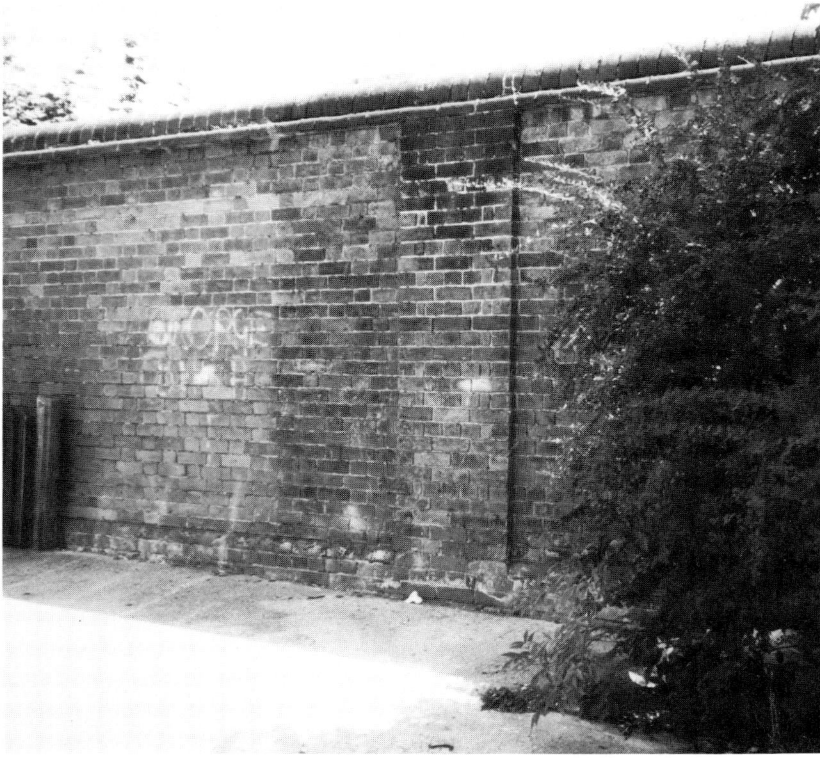

The Asylum wall in 1990

Pat and Rudi with best wishes
— Bernard.

A PROPER HOUSE

Bedford Lunatic Asylum (1812 – 1860)

by Bernard Cashman

"... it is expedient that further provision should be made for 'the care and maintenance of such persons and for the erecting proper houses for their reception'. . . ."

from "Wynn's Act": 1808

North Bedfordshire Health Authority

1992

By the same author:

PRIVATE CHARITY and the PUBLIC PURSE
– The development of Bedford General Hospital (1794-1988)

ISBN 0-9513626-2-3

Cover: Colour print of the Bedford asylum by T. Fisher c.1820
(Courtesy of County Record Office)

Photoset and printed by
Stanley L. Hunt (Printers) Ltd, Midland Road, Rushden, Northamptonshire

Contents

Acknowledgments

We are most grateful to the Marc Fitch Fund and to the Bedfordshire County Council for generous contributions towards the cost of publication of this book.

Our thanks are also due to Mr. Samuel Whitbread for permission to quote from the Whitbread correspondence. The Rt. Hon. William Waldegrave, MP has kindly furnished additional details about Samuel Whitbread II and the latter's son-in-law, Captain William Waldegrave, RN.

As always, the archivists and other staff of the County Record Office have been extremely helpful and patient in locating the source material. Much of it would not have come to light had it not been for the enterprise and persistence shown by James Collett-White, senior archivist, whose article on the Bedford asylum published in the *Bedfordshire Magazine* (see Bibliography) first captured my own interest. Nigel Lutt has not only contributed the account of John Harris's private asylum, which appears as Appendix III, but has been most energetic in tracking down certain of the illustrations.

We are very grateful to Chris Pickford, the county archivist, to John Turner, curator of the Bedford Museum and those others whose kind permission to reproduce illustrations is acknowledged in the appropriate place. David Bennett, district building officer, has been most helpful with expert advice and in the production of the plan showing the location of the asylum. Patricia Bell and Michael Shepherd have both contributed welcome encouragement and suggestions in the course of the writing of this book, and Margaret Allen has kindly undertaken the otherwise thankless task of preparing the index. The printers, Stanley L. Hunt Limited, have once more earned our thanks for their efficiency and expertise.

Finally, I wish to record my personal gratitude to David Brownridge, director of finance, for his very practical encouragement and support.

Foreword

by Michael Shepherd, CBE, MA, DM, FRCP, FRCPsych, DPM
Emeritus Professor of Epidemiological Psychiatry
Institute of Psychiatry, University of London

In their book, *The Hospital in History*,* Lindsay Granshaw and Roy Porter indicate some of the reasons for the current attention being paid by professional historians to the growth of hospitals in the recent and more remote past. Their concerns tend to focus on the various factors bearing on the role of the hospital as one of several institutions developed in response to a complex of social needs, taking its place alongside the school, the prison and the factory. Reviewing the field, Granshaw acknowledges the valuable contributions made by amateur historians, most of them medically qualified, who comment on the particular hospital with which they have been associated. These studies, she comments, "are very useful, providing much information, even if they may lack a sense of overall context".†

Possibly so, but a medical education conduces to an emphasis on factual information rather than on theoretical speculation. A surgical training is even more emphatic and the author of this monograph illustrates the merits of such an approach. Bernard Cashman is an orthopaedic surgeon who in retirement has engaged in local historical research and has written a history of Bedford General Hospital.‡ Here he enters choppier waters by providing an account of the Bedford Lunatic Asylum (1812-1860), one of the earliest to be built after the passage of the County Asylum Act of 1808. The many primary sources on which he has been able to draw include the asylum minutes, account books and visitors' reports; lists of patients, medical reports and journals; entries in contemporary newspapers and Quarter Sessions minutes; and the correspondence

---

* Granshaw, L. and Porter, R. (eds.), *The Hospital in History*, Routledge: London and New York, 1991.

† Granshaw, L., *op. cit.*, p. 12.

‡ Cashman, B., *Private Charity and the Public Purse*, N. Beds. Health Authority, 1988.

of the redoubtable Samuel Whitbread, the prime mover in the creation of the asylum.

The picture emerging from this grass-roots inquiry is that of a mosaic depicting what the author calls "the birth, life and death" of an institution. By and large he allows the facts to speak for themselves and his commentary is chronological rather than interpretative. Nonetheless, the work casts a long shadow over the modern movement towards the de-institutionalization and the community care of the mentally ill. As such it is of more than historical interest.

Introduction

The Bedford asylum in Ampthill Road was opened for the reception of pauper and criminal lunatics in 1812. It was only the second to have been built in England in accordance with the Act of Parliament of 1808, which permitted, or even encouraged, counties to create such institutions – Nottingham was first off the mark in 1811. The asylum was the fifth of Bedford's most important public institutions which were either constructed or rebuilt during the turbulent period which began with the start of the French Revolution in 1789 and ended with Napoleon's defeat at Waterloo in 1815. They were, in chronological order:

(a) The House of Industry, the town workhouse, built in 1794 – it became, ultimately, the North Wing of Bedford General Hospital;
(b) Bedford Prison, rebuilt in 1801. Further major reconstruction was started in 1991, nearly 200 years later;
(c) Bedford Infirmary, the voluntary hospital, eventually the South Wing of the district general hospital, created in 1948;
(d) The Town Bridge, a vitally important river crossing, was rebuilt in 1811; and
(e) The County Lunatic Asylum (1812), which is the subject of this book.

The prime mover in all five was Samuel Whitbread II (1764-1815), a man of extraordinary talents who, had it not been for his fiery temperament, might have attained the highest political position in the land. This is an account of how the Bedford asylum came to be built, of its progress through the first half of the 19th century, and of its closure in 1860 when the demand for its facilities outstripped its resources, and the Three Counties asylum was opened.

It is said that there are several basic questions that need to be answered by those who, for whatever reasons, undertake studies such as this; John Pickstone, for example, has written that:

> ". . . there is no set agenda for medical historians, except to pursue questions of general significance that are also feasible in the particular. The usual historical enquiries: why here?, why then?, why in this form? apply easily to institutions and other local phenomena."*

The population of Bedfordshire at the beginning of the 19th century numbered about 63,000; only Rutland and Monmouth had fewer. Most were occupied on the land, or in cottage industries such as lace-making. There was a thriving trade in corn, which was transported by water on the river, the Great Ouse, to the East Anglian ports in exchange for the coal that came back along the same route.

In 1806, in the face of the growing social, economic and humanitarian problems of lunacy, the House of Commons appointed a select committee to make recommendations on the subject. It was at a time when the madness of the king, George III, was producing major constitutional and political difficulties which were to be resolved only by the establishment of the Regency in 1811.

Samuel Whitbread was Bedford's MP at the time and a member of the select committee, one of whose earliest moves was to conduct a nationwide survey; a questionnaire was directed to all the counties of England – how many pauper lunatics and how many idiots (mentally handicapped) were living there? Possibly from civic pride or, more probably, from an uneasy (and, in the end, justifiable) suspicion that it was going to cost them, the county of Bedford submitted a nil return; no such persons were to be found in their parishes.

They were not alone in their negative response, but in its final report, the committee reached the conclusion that a county asylum for Bedfordshire alone would not be viable, and proposed that four counties combine for the purpose, the institution being situated at Oxford. Why, therefore, was it built at Bedford, and why so soon after the passage of the Act of Parliament which made it possible?

---

* Pickstone, John V., *Social History of Medicine*, Vol. 2, 2, p. 198.

I believe that the answer to Professor Pickstone's first two questions rests largely on Samuel Whitbread's personality and career. As will be seen, his domination of the committee of visiting justices was almost total. It was Whitbread who appointed the staff, selected the furniture and equipment and winkled out suitable patients from the reluctant parish officers. He placed great reliance on the advice given to him by Thomas Dunston, master of St. Luke's Hospital, established in London in 1751, whom he had heard giving evidence to the select committee, and the initial organisation and conduct of the Bedford asylum were modelled fairly closely on that older prototype, although on a much reduced scale.

Three years after the pattern had been established, Samuel Whitbread killed himself. The affairs of the asylum continued on the pragmatic course he had set, the numbers of inmates mounting steadily and the design and the limited scale of the building showing increasing signs of inadequacy.

The governance of the institution was initially entrusted by Whitbread to the inappropriate hands of a house-painter, whose appearance, and that of his wife, had pleased him. With the appointment of Dr. Joseph Thackeray as (non-resident) physician, however, the supremacy of medical responsibility in the treatment of the patients was firmly established. That process had been started by Thackeray's predecessor, the otherwise ineffectual Dr. Yeats (and then it was from what seems to have been mainly a matter of personal pride).

Important changes were made after the Bedford and all other county asylums came under the scrutiny of the Commissioners in Lunacy who were appointed under the terms of the 1845 legislation. The remaining years of the Bedford asylum saw the final abolition of crude physical restraints – the chains, handcuffs and strait-jackets applied to the more "difficult" patients – and the appointment of a resident medical superintendent.

Despite the provision of some additional accommodation, the building was bursting at the seams by the 1850s; from housing only 24 patients in 1812, there were 270 by 1853 and, four years later, 323. Many of these were drawn from counties other than Bedfordshire, and when a survey produced plans to redevelop on the existing site, the prospective cost was such as to make the decision to move to a new building on a different site inevitable.

A union with two adjoining counties, those of Hertford and Huntingdon, was created for the purpose, and despite some local opposition, notably from the Borough of Bedford, the Three Counties Asylum, now Fairfield Hospital, was built at Arlesey, the capital and revenue costs being shared *pro rata* according to an agreed formula. A fourth county, Cambridgeshire, might well have been included, but the negotiations broke down when the other three insisted on the appointment of an independent arbitrator to decide on the proportion of the contribution to be made by Cambridge.

It seems to me that any account of the birth, life and death of an institution has much in common with the biography of an individual, and I have kept to a chronological format. While attempting to meet the historians' terms, I hope also to have produced a portrait of the Bedford lunatic asylum which will be of interest to those whose curiosity about the residues of the past which surround most of us matches my own.

B.C.

CHAPTER ONE

The Select Committee of 1807

During the second half of the 18th century the need for reform of the ways in which the insane were treated was brought to the attention of the general public by a number of events. Kathleen Jones* has referred, for example, to the revision of the vagrancy laws concerning dangerous lunatics in 1744; this was followed nearly 20 years later by publication of the details of the awful conditions in many private asylums ("madhouses"), where those mentally ill patients were confined who could afford, or whose friends and relatives had the means, to pay for their keep.

Under the 1744 Act, lunatic paupers were exempted from the range of punishments and deterrents applied to those vagrants who appeared to be sane. The law allowed the latter to be arrested by anybody, taken before a magistrate and imprisoned in a House of Correction with hard labour. (The informant was given a reward of five shillings.)

Two Justices of the Peace were now required to issue a warrant to the parish officers, i.e. the overseers of the poor, the churchwardens and the constables, for the "lunatick or mad person" to be locked up in some secure place and if they thought necessary, to be kept in chains for his own protection, or for the safety of others. This restraint was to be continued for as long as the disordered state of mind was deemed to have persisted and, as Jones observes, the "secure place" was usually a gaol.

A local example of this procedure was provided by an order signed at the quarter session court on October 23rd 1799 in respect of Elizabeth Stodge:

> "Bedfordshire: To the constable, churchwardens and overseers of the poor of the parish of Arlesey in the said county of Bedford.

---

* K. Jones, *A history of the mental health services 1972* – see Bibliography.

> Whereas it hath been proved before us two of the justices of our lord the king assigned to keep the peace within the said county [and] upon the oaths of William Tristram and William Robertson both of the parish of Arlesey in the county aforesaid yeomen . . . that Elizabeth Stodge of Arlesey frequently goeth at large in the said parish of Arlesey and . . . is by lunacy so far disordered in her senses that she is dangerous to be permitted to go abroad and that her legal settlement is in the said parish of Arlesey, these are therefore to authorise and require you and every one of you to cause the said Elizabeth Stodge to be kept safely locked up . . . [in her own house] . . . or any other house as the churchwardens and overseers shall think the most convenient allowing her proper maintenance at the expense of the said parish and that the said house be a secure place and the said Elizabeth Stodge is to be kept locked up only so long as such lunacy or disorder shall continue and no longer. . . ."

Such was the shortage of suitable accommodation in the parishes that overseers often sent insane paupers to private institutions at the public expense. Payment for their maintenance out of the public purse was, as might have been expected, by no means lavish, and that was reflected in the poor quality of the treatment they received.

The cost of maintenance in prison or in private was to be recovered from the individual's estate, or by seizure and sale of his property, over and above whatever was considered necessary for the support of his family. If he had nothing, the cost would fall on the parish, as with any other pauper; in that case it was in the interest of the parish in which he was apprehended, if he were not legally "settled" there, to get him transferred to the place where he belonged.

To the cost of maintenance was added that of curing him – even though no effective treatment other than restraint was generally available. Even if medical certification had been required (and it wasn't) registration of doctors was not introduced until more than a century later; in any case, recognition of madness as a form of illness was still encumbered by notions of demonic possession or of retribution for past sins.

The local magistrates, who had the responsibility for deciding that someone was insane, how he or she should be handled and for how long, were not necessarily equipped with either medical or legal training, and the law still gave little protection to the mentally ill against unscrupulous gaolers or avaricious relatives.

The lot of patients detained in private asylums was often little better than for those in gaol. The publicity surrounding some cases of wrongful detention in such places caused general alarm and gave rise, eventually, to the Act of Parliament of 1774 for the regulation of all private madhouses (14 Geo.III c.9).

The Act established commissioners, elected from the Royal College of Physicians, who were to visit all such houses and report on the condition of the patients there, and to be responsible for licensing them. Outside the metropolitan area, however, these duties became the responsibility of two justices and a physician who were nominated at Quarter Sessions.

No private institutions existed in Bedfordshire until Springfield House was opened by John Harris in Kempston in 1837, and a private asylum in Hoxton was favoured by some of the overseers in the rural parishes before that time.

It was not until about 1788 that the general public became aware of serious constitutional problems ahead arising from the illness of the king, George III, who had attempted to subdue the Commons and, in the words of Trevelyan, "to take back the patronage of the Crown into the royal hands".* It is now suggested that the king was suffering from *porphyria*, a fairly rare metabolic disorder, but at the time it was generally assumed that his manic outbursts were the result of mental illness. Although attacks had occurred in the past, they were not so severe as the one in 1788 which rendered him incapable of attending to his royal duties; the Prince of Wales (later the Prince Regent) told his friends, for example, of a physical attack made on him by his father because of some imagined insult.

The madness of the king now became a significant issue in the political struggle between the Whig opposition, led by Charles James Fox and the Tory government, at whose head was William Pitt the Younger, installed by, and retaining the support of the king.

The Prince, however, favoured the Whigs and if the king's illness were to be declared incurable, the establishment of a Regency was inevitable. And so the battle was joined.

---

* Trevelyan, G. M. *A shortened history of England,* 1942.

The king's own doctors doubted that he would recover quickly and naturally, they gained the support of the Whig faction, which included Samuel Whitbread II (whose father was not, however, to hand over his seat in the House of Commons to his son until the following year).

Pitt then engaged Dr. Francis Willis, the proprietor of a private madhouse who "was certain that he could restore the king's sanity within a few months". Willis was a former vicar of Wapping who had taken up medical practice and had developed methods of treatment which, though they horrified some observers, were considered justifiable by others who did not relish the prospect of a government headed by Fox.

Kathleen Jones quotes Countess Harcourt:

> ". . . he was no longer treated as a human being. His body was immediately encased in a machine which left it no liberty of motion. He was sometimes chained to a staple and . . . kept in subjection by menacing and violent language."

Such was the public concern that a select committee of the House of Commons was appointed to enquire into the king's condition. His own physician, Dr. Warren, had maintained that there was no improvement and accused Dr. Willis of issuing misleading progress reports.

The committee, which included such notables as Lord North, William Wilberforce (later the reformer of the slave trade), Lord Grenville and both Fox and the playwright, Sheridan, reached the conclusion that the king was indeed incurable. A bill to establish a Regency was introduced and was about to be read for the third time, when the royal patient staged a sudden recovery, and the legislation was shelved.

"Madness," says Jones, "had become a respectable malady . . . one which was susceptible to treatment and capable of cure." No matter that the treatment included the application of hot irons, strait-jackets and other methods and instruments more appropriate to the torture chamber.

In 1801, the king suffered a relapse and Dr. Willis and his sons applied the same measures; again their patient recovered – but not for long. Further maniacal attacks occurred and the Regency Bill

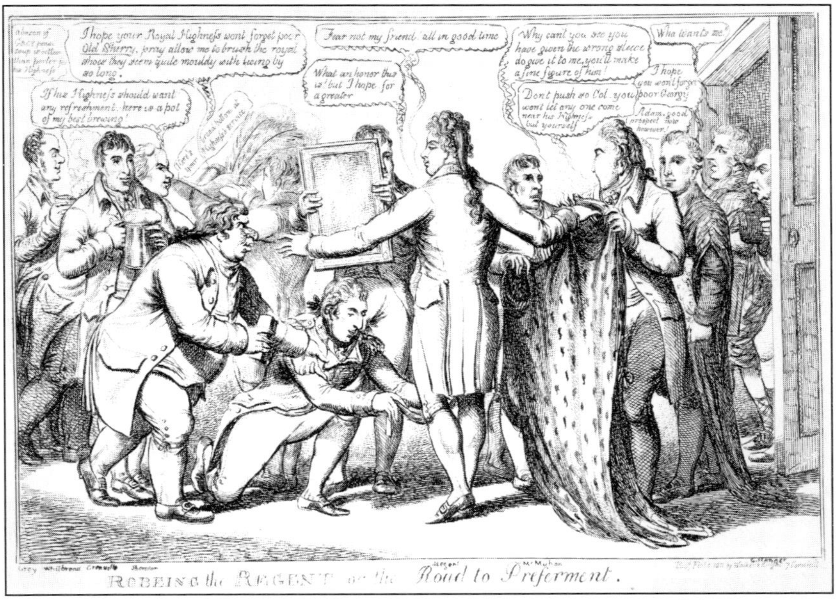
I hope your Royal Highness wont forget poor Old Sherry, pray allow me to brush the royal shoes they seem quite mouldy with being by so long.
If his Highness should want any refreshment, here is a pot of my best brewing!
Fear not my friend, all in good time
What an honor this is! but I hope for a greater
Why cant you see you have given the wrong sleeve do give it to me, you'll make a fine figure of him!
Who wants me!
I hope you wont forget poor Georgy
Dont push so Col. you wont let any one come near his Highness but yourself
Adam, good prospect now however!
Grey Whitbread Grenville Sheridan
Regent
McMahon
ROBEING the REGENT or the Road to Preferment.

Political print by Charles Williams, published 1811. Courtesy of the Trustees of the British Museum

was taken from the shelf and dusted off. (It was to become law in 1811.)

By this time, Samuel Whitbread had entered Parliament as the Member for Bedford and had already established his reputation as "England's leading radical MP, fearless and dominating" (Cole).

In 1794 he had steered through the Commons the bill which established the House of Industry, the workhouse for the town, and in 1801, as a leading light among the magistrates (he served the Biggleswade division until his death in 1815), Whitbread was an important member of the committee responsible for rebuilding the County Gaol. His father died in 1796 and on his son's shoulders were heaped, *inter alia*, all the arrangements for building, staffing and managing the Bedford Infirmary, the voluntary hospital which ultimately became the South Wing of Bedford General Hospital – the North Wing developed from the sick wards of the House of Industry.*

---

* Details of this aspect of Whitbread's remarkable career are contained in the present author's history of Bedford General Hospital, *Private Charity and the Public Purse* – see bibliography.

From about 1805, Whitbread became a favourite subject for inclusion in the political cartoons which proliferated in the early nineteenth century; he appeared in satires by such noted artists as Gillray, Charles Williams, Rowlandson and the Cruikshanks. Dennis Cole* identified 66 such prints in the British Library in which he figured prominently, usually as the fierce scourge of wrongdoers, particularly those in high places.

Samuel Whitbread was noted as the proposer of measures for regulating the wages of labourers and for the education of the poor. His support for the principles (but not the practice) of the French Revolution and his outspoken opposition to the declaration of war on Napoleon after the latter's escape from Elba earned him the hostility of the Tory faction.

On Pitt's death in 1806 Lord Grenville was invited to form a broadly based government – the "Ministry of all the Talents" – which was to last for little more than one year. Charles James Fox, who was already a dying man, became Foreign Secretary and Lord Grey, Whitbread's brother-in-law (and a fellow Foxite Whig), was made First Lord of the Admiralty.

Whitbread's exclusion from office was a shattering blow. He wrote to Grey:

> "My constituents received me with looks of surprise, and . . . stupidly supposed that whenever the turn [to a Whig government] should happen I should be among the first wanted. . . ."

After this time, it appears that he became disillusioned with national politics and turned increasingly to his Bedfordshire interests, much to the advantage of the county. One more major effort was needed from him in the House of Commons and he rose to the challenge with his usual vigour. In 1806, Whitbread was appointed to the Select Committee which was to "enquire into the State of the Criminal and Pauper Lunatics in England and Wales, and of the Laws relating thereto . . .".

The select committee of 1806 was set up in response to persistent representations by Sir George Onesiphorous Paul, a Gloucestershire magistrate who, Scull† says, "bombarded the Home Office with

---

* See bibliography.

† A. Scull, *Museums of madness* – see bibliography.

complaints about the anomalies in the existing laws dealing with lunatics". Paul urged the establishment of a system of tax-supported asylums; he had been frustrated in his attempts to establish one based on charity and associated with the Gloucester Infirmary.

The membership of the select committee included Samuel Whitbread and his friend Sir Samuel Romilly; George Rose, sponsor of the Friendly Societies Act of 1793 and William Wilberforce, who campaigned successfully against the slave trade.* The committee sat for some months and on July 15th 1807 its final report was published. This report formed the basis on which legislation, in the form of the "Act for the better Cure and Maintenance of Lunatics, being Paupers or Criminals in England" [43 Geo.III c.96] was enacted.

The report, with its eight appendices, paints a vivid picture of the spirit of the times and the wretched physical conditions to which these poor creatures were subjected. It is not difficult to imagine the effect on Whitbread, preoccupied as he was by what must have seemed an end to his ability to influence the great affairs of state.

But the nation's loss was Bedford's gain; what he learned while serving on that committee was to produce a county asylum which was only the second to have been built in the kingdom.

The report† begins with a description of the existing laws respecting the care of criminal and pauper lunatics. In the case of the criminally insane, the only law relating to them was Geo.III c.94, whereby evidence that someone on trial for treason, felony or murder was insane at the time of the offence could enable the Court to commit him into custody – whether the jury found him guilty or not – "until His Majesty's pleasure be known".

Since the Act had been passed six years earlier, no fewer than 37 people had been detained in this way; those of them who were paupers were of necessity kept in prison at the county's expense. The numbers were expected to increase, particularly "if the parishes upon whom the burden of their maintenance would otherwise fall should ... be enabled to throw that expense on the county at large".

---

* Scull quotes Sidney Smith, the noted wit, as referring to one of Wilberforce's favourite organisations, the Society for the Suppression of Vice, as "a society for suppressing the vices of persons whose income does not exceed £500 per annum".

† Report on the select committee on the state of lunatics 1807; British Library.

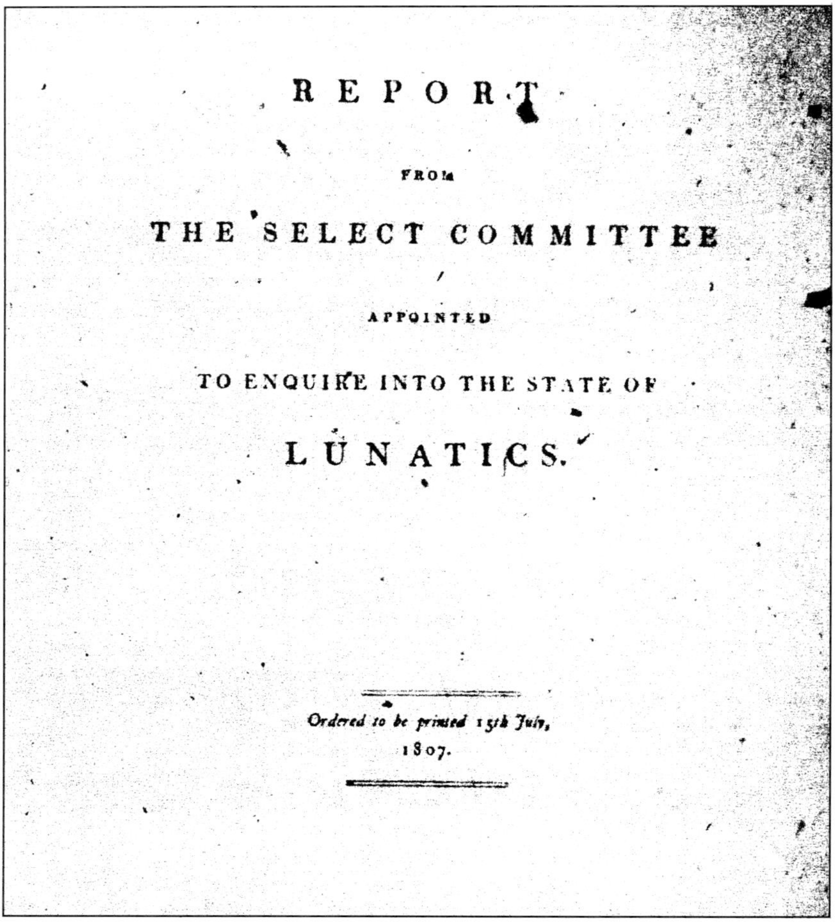

REPORT

FROM

THE SELECT COMMITTEE

APPOINTED

TO ENQUIRE INTO THE STATE OF

LUNATICS.

Ordered to be printed 15th July,
1807.

Thus, the first concern of the committee was to answer a question of perennial interest – who would have to pay for whatever solution they produced?

After hearing evidence from Paul and others about the damaging effects on criminal lunatics of their confinement in common prisons, the committee recommended, for those detained under the provisions of the Act, a special asylum. If a prisoner there had insufficient funds for his maintenance, i.e. was a pauper as well as being a criminal, the magistrates of the county could order the parish where he was last settled to pay for him.

The select committee then heard verbal evidence from Sir G. O. Paul on the subject of pauper lunatics who had committed no criminal offences. When he was asked if the necessary attendance could be supplied as cheaply in a gaol as in special accommodation, he replied that "it probably could".

In response to a question as to whether he had observed the manner in which lunatics were kept in the parishes, Paul replied that he had often seen such poorhouses but that in no instance had he seen them kept with any regard to their cure. He had seen some who were not in poorhouses:

> ". . . fastened to the leg of a table in a dwelling house . . . others chained to a post in an outhouse: and in one instance I witnessed a man chained in an uninhabited ruin and food brought to him from his relations, living at a quarter of a mile distance."

Paul was asked about the cost of maintenance in a "proper house" for the reception of lunatics and he produced figures which showed that the greater the number of patients, the lower the cost per head. But he was careful to draw attention to the effects of inflation – he had made his calculations in 1796 when, for example, 7s.6d. (the cost per head of 67 patients) would now, in 1807, be the equivalent of 9s.6d.

Oral evidence was next given by Thomas Dunston, the master of St. Luke's Hospital. He had been in the post for more than 25 years, and Samuel Whitbread, always ready to acknowledge the expert, was greatly impressed. St. Luke's had been established in London in 1751; it was a charitable institution of high repute and, says Scull, represented "a major attempt to assert medical control over the problem of insanity". The officers and staff at the hospital included a non-resident physician, surgeon and secretary, an apothecary and his wife, and a master and matron.

The average number of patients was 300, and on the waiting list, 640.

Dunston said that before joining St. Luke's, he had been employed at Bedlam (Bethlem Hospital, established in 1377).

> "Q – In what capacity was you at Bedlam?"
> "A – As keeper for 7 or 8 years."

He was subjected to detailed questioning about the dimensions of the hospital and the committee subsequently recommended that the ideal asylum should contain as many patients as possible, but not more than 300.

Dunston was asked about the food supplied to the patients at St. Luke's and gave the following typical bill of fare:

> *Breakfast:* Water gruel with bread, butter and salt.
> *Dinner:* On four days of the week – meat, with "the best table beer".
> Monday, Wednesday and Saturday – broth.
> Variation of this diet for sick patients took the form of "beef-tea, broth, sago and wine etc.".

On the matter of treatment, he thought that about three patients in 20 required coercion; they were the ones who were disposed to injure themselves or others. Dunston agreed with a suggestion that a large proportion of patients "by a firm and uniform management . . . become tractable". Idiots (i.e. the mentally handicapped) were not admitted to St. Luke's Hospital.

> "Q – Have you found any advantage from the cold baths . . .?"
> "A – Yes; by washing and keeping them clean in warm weather."

That concluded the evidence given by Thomas Dunston. It will be noted later how closely, mainly at Whitbread's insistence, the Bedford asylum was to be modelled on the St. Luke's pattern.

John Nash, the distinguished architect, said that he had turned his thoughts to the construction of a lunatic asylum and had drawn up plans for such buildings (by subscription) at Hereford, Exeter and one not yet completed at Gloucester. He gave his opinion of the probable cost of building an asylum for 50 patients in London; it would have, for example, walls two bricks deep, wards 12′ × 10′, "floors and partitions filled with sawdust, to prevent the communication of sound", and two water-closets in each division of a ward.

The cost of such a building would, he estimated, amount to £7,760.

There can be little doubt that Samuel Whitbread was studying all the proceedings with his usual care. St. Luke's Hospital had been designed by George Dance (the architect responsible for Newgate

Prison). Scull quotes John Connolly: "... the architects of this period appear to have had regard solely to the safe-keeping of the inmates and the buildings resembled prisons rather than hospitals for the cure of insanity." When the time came for decision on his home ground, Whitbread turned to John Wing, who had designed and built the House of Industry, the Infirmary, and Bedford Gaol.

Dr. Francis Willis, whose involvement in the treatment of King George has been noted, gave verbal evidence to the committee. In his opinion, a house for the reception of lunatics ought to be visited daily by a "medical person". Each patient required a separate plan of treatment. Warm baths might be useful, but cold ones were very seldom needed.

"Q – Are you of opinion that, in such a house, it is necessary the convalescent should be separated from the other patients?"

"A – I do not think in general that such a separation is called for, not having found ... any disadvantage arise from the want of it."

"Q – Do you consider it to be at all disadvantageous that a lunatic should be removed to a distance from his friends?"

"A – I do not conceive it to be disadvantageous in general, in some instances even *advantageous*."

Dr. Halliday, in a letter to the chairman (Mr. Charles Watkin Williams Wynn) referred to the treatment of the mentally handicapped in Suffolk. Many were in workhouses as common paupers, but in some parishes the "poor idiot" was allowed to stay with his family and on the parish. But at one time, some farmers pretended that they had a secret remedy for madness and would take on the "unhappy beings" (with their funds) so that the farmer got his rent as well as a supply of free labour!

The select committee then considered a plan whereby the kingdom would be divided into districts in which it would be appropriate to build county asylums. They reached the conclusion that the optimum size of population for such a district was half a million.*

* This corresponds closely with the maximum permitted size of a health district under the reorganisation of the NHS in 1982.

Apart from the metropolis, the only single counties with populations surpassing that figure were Yorkshire (858,892) and its ancient rival, Lancashire (672,731). The committee therefore proposed a total of 16 districts, No. 12 of which would combine the counties of:

Oxford (109,620), Berks. (109,215), Bucks. (107,444) and Bedford (63,393). The asylum for this combined district should, they suggest, be sited at *Oxford*.

Of all the counties, only Rutland and Monmouth were smaller, in terms of population, than Bedfordshire, but that was unlikely to have deterred Whitbread, particularly in view of the conclusion in the report that the building ought to be so sited as to be easily accessible to the "best medical assistance". He was still actively concerned in the management of the Bedford Infirmary (which was largely his creation), and he must have known that any subsequent legislation following the committee's report would be permissive rather than prescriptive, and that Bedford would be able to build its own asylum.

Furthermore:

> ". . . in all cases it may be desirable to allow the addition of an establishment for persons of a superior class to be defrayed by themselves; and for those in a state of distress, though not actually parish paupers, to be maintained by charitable subscription."

Here, then, was an opportunity to combine the public purse with private charity, and Samuel Whitbread, still smarting from his disappointment at his exclusion from government, was not slow to grasp it.

The County Asylums Act of 1808 (48 Geo.III c.96) was piloted through both Houses of Parliament without difficulty;* it reflected closely the recommendations of the select committee and included detailed specifications for the construction of asylums by those counties which chose to implement it. It was "expedient" – but not compulsory – that proper houses be erected for the care and maintenance of "lunatics and other insane persons", and it was for

* It became known as "Wynn's Act" after the chairman of the select committee.

the Justices of the Peace to decide whether or not to combine with other counties for the purpose.

The building should be ". . . as far as conveniently may be, fixed upon an airy and healthy situation with a good supply of water and which may afford the probability of the vicinity of constant medical assistance".

Separate wards for males and females, and for convalescent and incurable patients were specified, as were day rooms and airing grounds; there should be "dry and airy cells for the lunatics of every description".

Kathleen Jones* says that, ". . . the importance of the Act lies primarily in the conception of treatment of a non-deterrent type as a public responsibility and in an attempt to deal with the root cause rather than with the symptoms of anti-social behaviour".

The justices could nominate and appoint visiting magistrates to superintend the building and management of such institutions and to report back to the Court of Quarter Sessions. Contracts were to be entered into "at the most reasonable rates and with the most responsible persons". The expenses arising from the execution of the Act were to be met out of special or ordinary county rates, and the rate-payers of the county could inspect the books at reasonable times.

Justices of the Peace connected with the execution of the Act were not allowed to have a financial interest in any contracts in which the asylum was concerned. (A similar restriction was applied to the business interests of the directors of the House of Industry and their successors.) They were authorised to issue warrants, on application by parish overseers, for "the conveyance of any lunatic, insane person or dangerous idiot who may be chargeable to such parish" to the asylum, to be kept there until a majority of the visiting justices thought them fit for discharge. The parishes were to be charged a weekly sum judged suitable for "maintenance, medicine, clothing and care".

Not surprisingly, the effect of that sting in the tail was to discourage many overseers from providing the Bedford asylum with

* See bibliography.

inmates, once Whitbread and his colleagues had got it built and staffed and equipped. Indeed, a preliminary survey in Bedfordshire had produced a nil return – there were, it seemed, no pauper lunatics anywhere in the county, not even in the area (Biggleswade) where Whitbread was a magistrate!

An amendment to Wynn's Act* was passed in 1811; overseers were now bound, under pain of a heavy fine, to give information of all insane persons in their area, and JPs were equally obliged to send those in poverty or who showed criminal tendencies to the asylum. The medical superintendent of every asylum had to make regular returns at least annually to the justices at general or quarter sessions, stating the condition of the patients under his care; in the light of those reports they could direct the discharge of any persons who might appear (to them) "to be no longer fit objects to remain therein".

---

* 51 Geo.III c.79.

CHAPTER TWO

Foundations: 1808-12

On October 5th 1808, the magistrates, who included Lord St. John, William Wilshere and Samuel Whitbread, met and ordered that a notice be placed in the *Northampton Mercury*:

> ". . . of their taking into consideration at the next Quarter Sessions the expediency and propriety of providing a lunatic asylum or house for the reception of lunatics and other insane persons."

A small committee was appointed to superintend the building and management of the asylum; it consisted of John, Duke of Bedford, the Earl of Upper Ossory and Samuel Whitbread. As Fulford* has said of him, ". . . with the Duke of Bedford, Whitbread enjoyed powers which might well have been envied by a modern county council". There was no doubt about which architect would be engaged.

John Wing (1756-1826) was the son of a John Wing of Hallerton, in Leicestershire. The family moved to Bedfordshire in the 1780s, the father having acquired a stone-quarry at Totternhoe. The son took over the quarry in due course and "... soon became the leading architect and builder of the county".† Wing made a number of monuments in Bedford, Flitton, Henlow, Sandy etc., and designed and built the House of Industry in 1796, Bedford Gaol in 1801, and the Bedford Infirmary in 1803. He was now in his second term of office as mayor of the town.

In April 1809, John Wing produced his first set of plans for an asylum of 100 inmates, but the estimated cost was such as to cause the committee to draw back. They called for a new plan for one of

* Roger Fulford – see Bibliography.
† *The Dictionary of British Architects*, p. 906 – see Bibliography.

only 40 patients, "... but without destroying the uniformity of the building". Wing quickly obliged, and produced a plan and elevation "with the addition of ... stone rustic ornaments and stone strings". The total cost, including Yorkshire stone coping to the walls would amount to £9,585 – to be paid by quarterly instalments of £500.

The plans were agreed and John Miller, the chairman of the committee, was deputed to negotiate with the Duke of Bedford for a suitable site for the asylum. On April 20th he wrote to the Duke:

> "... permit me to inform your Grace that Mr. Wing pointed out a close belonging to your Grace, now or late in the occupation of Mrs. Meacock which from its high situation, proper aspect for maniacs, fit distance from the Infirmary [these terms are a direct quotation from the Act] and other circumstances, I cannot but concur with Mr. Wing in thinking the best spot. . . ."

There were three acres in the close, but only half of it would be needed for the building. It was intended that the front of the asylum would face the Ampthill Road "on the opposite side to where the Infirmary is and at 300 yards distance from it".*

The field was eventually purchased for £345, which included three years' rental of the land while the building was under construction. During that time, Samuel Whitbread was far from idle; he undertook personal charge of the arrangements for the management, the staffing, the furniture and the equipment of the institution. Thomas Dunston, the manager of St. Luke's Hospital, had impressed him by the evidence he had given to the Select Committee, and Whitbread was to rely heavily on his advice and practical help in getting the Bedford asylum started.

Overall control of the asylum was vested in a committee of visiting magistrates. Those appointed in January 1809 included the Duke of Bedford, the Earl of Upper Ossory, Francis Pym, Samuel Whitbread and his friend William Wilshere. The chairman was John Miller.

On April 8th 1812, a letter from Samuel Whitbread was read to the visiting magistrates, as he was unable to attend on that day:

The asylum was now ready to be handed over to the county.

---

* The chosen site was in the close now bounded by Offa, Mabel and Muswell Roads.

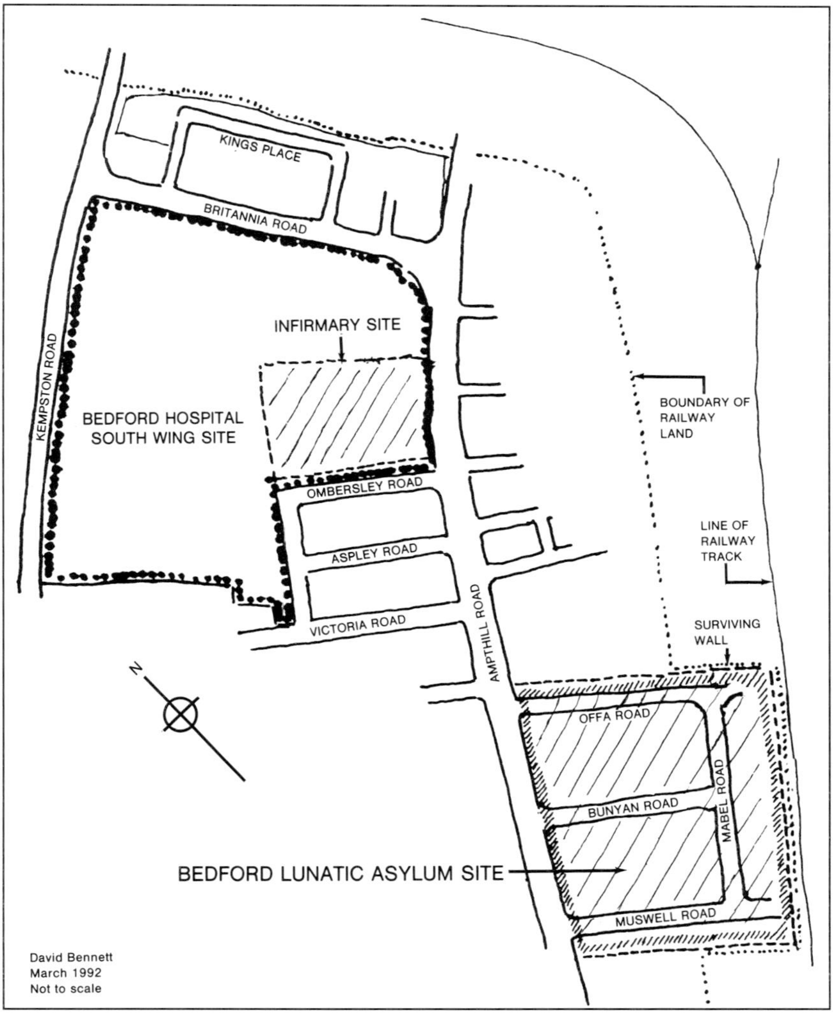

Part of Bedford in 1991 showing the former site of the Asylum and Infirmary. Drawn by David Bennett

". . . I went over the building with him [John Wing] the other day . . . I should hope by timely exertion there could be no doubt of its being made available to the county by midsummer next."

Some items were still lacking, including beds; the pattern for these would be obtained from the maker of the beds at St. Luke's as would be the case for the grates and fireguards. Two of the boilers at the

Infirmary had been taken down because they were too large for the establishment – they might serve for the asylum.

As for furniture for the staff, i.e. the master and matron (as at the workhouse): ". . . I should think in all probility *[sic]* would be a married pair." For levelling of the ground and planting a kitchen garden, which was to be outside the asylum walls, he recommended "the man who has the care of the Infirmary gardens".

Whitbread had taken advice about medical cover and it had been agreed locally that William Leech, who held the combined post at the Infirmary of house surgeon, apothecary and hospital secretary, might, for an additional salary, attend the asylum in a similar capacity. Leech had ably discharged his duties at the Infirmary and "the patients in the asylum will not be of a description to require the same species of unremitting attention during the 24 hours". Drugs could be provided initially from the stores at the Infirmary – "upon proper payment being made".

On the recommendations of "Mr. Dunster" [Thomas Dunston], Whitbread had already interviewed two applicants with their wives for the posts of master and matron. Either would be competent and "one of whom I think would be very eligible, and his wife even more so".

The first, a Mr. Jackson, was about 40 years old, and an assistant at a Foundation school near London. Whitbread found him to be an orderly, decent-looking man who wrote a good hand "but the appearance of his wife, on whom so much must depend . . . was not exactly such as pleased me".

The other applicant was William Pither, "a young man not 30 years of age of simple unassuming appearance, and his wife with all the characteristics of a person fitted for the situation". Pither was now a painter by trade, having been called to attend a tradesman of that description who was deranged and "for whom he conducted the business during his indisposition".*

Both applicants were willing to undertake the office for a salary of 60 guineas per annum – exclusive of board and the use of the furniture. Another applicant of suitable appearance had been

* Whitbread's acceptance of this as adequate experience for the onerous tasks ahead gives some support to the views of those of his contemporaries who felt that he was sometimes given to over-hasty judgments.

interviewed, but he was unmarried, which Whitbread considered a conclusive objection. It is evident from the letters written by Jackson that he was under the impression that he had been offered the job, but when the true position was made clear, Jackson withdrew his application on the grounds that he "declined entering into any contest with so many competitions for the situation".

William Pither was duly appointed in April 1812 under the title of "governor" – the term "master", with its poor-law connotations, having been discarded. His wife, Mary, whose fitness for the post had so impressed Samuel Whitbread, was appointed matron, and the couple were granted removal expenses of five pounds.

Attention now turned to the important matter of medical staffing. It had been intended to appoint William Leech, the house surgeon at the infirmary, to the post of surgeon-in-attendance, subject to the agreement of the governors of that institution. However, one of the two (honorary) surgeons at the hospital had written to the committee:

> "Mr. John Pulley presents his most respectful compliments to the magistrates of the County of Bedford and begs leave to offer his services without emolument as Surgeon to the intended lunatic asylum."

His colleague, Charles Short, made a similar offer and both were gratefully accepted. Leech was not left out, though, and the title of his appointment was changed to that of "medical-attendant-in-ordinary".

One man was decidedly unhappy at what must have seemed to the justices a quite adequate arrangement for medical care. Dr. Yeats, the first and solitary physician to the Bedford Infirmary, had written to Whitbread as early as December 1808, giving his views on how the asylum ought to be designed and managed; his letter had been ignored.

Grant David Yeats was born into a colonial family in Florida in 1773. He moved to England and graduated in medicine from Oxford in 1793, being already established in his practice in Bedford when the infirmary was opened in 1803. His appointment as physician to the hospital appears to have been unopposed, and he quickly busied himself with the rules and regulations of the establishment (which did not endear him to his colleagues). Yeats became involved in several heated arguments on medical matters and leaned heavily on Samuel Whitbread for support.*

In 1806, the Duke of Bedford went to Ireland as Lord Lieutenant, and Dr. Yeats accompanied him as his personal physician. The Rev. Philip Hunt, Rector of St. Paul's Church, was the Duke's chaplain on that occasion.

In 1808, Yeats had written to Samuel Whitbread, saying that he had been reading the Act, which gave the county "considerable latitude in the dimensions of the proposed asylum" which ought to be proportioned to the number of patients likely to be admitted. According to the enquiry which, he wrote, Whitbread had instituted, there were "as many lunatics in the county as there were parishes", i.e. 147.

Not as many places as that would be required (an opinion in which Yeats was, for once, correct). Many would be "restored as reasonable members to society". Their present state was in his opinion owing to neglect. Mania was not, he asserted, like the physical ["corporal"] diseases to which the poor were subjected, with their mode of living, exposure to all kinds of weather and laborious work.

He had acquired a copy of a plan for an asylum in Glasgow, and he offered to send the plan to Whitbread; it was, he said, "a very ingenious design resembling Blackburn's penitentiary houses".†

This offer was not, it seems, taken up. He made further proposals in 1812, by which time the recruitment of the honorary medical staff of the asylum appeared to have been completed – without a physician, and more specifically, without Dr. Yeats. In September, he wrote to "his illustrious patron", the Duke of Bedford (and sent a copy to Whitbread).

In his letter, Yeats complained that he had suggested a plan "... whereby the physician was remunerated without any burden falling on the public purse". Payment would be made to the physician by such patients as were able to afford it, i.e. those who were, in his words, "above the class of paupers.... Your Grace will see from the turn of my letter (enclosed) how far I was disposed to render professional assistance to the asylum". Whitbread had replied to the

---

* *Private Charity and the Public Purse*, see Bibliography.

† William Blackburn, architect (1750-1790) – a pioneer of prison design.

effect that the plan would probably be adopted at some future date, but had not referred to it again.

"I have felt hurt," Yeats wrote, "that an institution *purely medical in all its branches** should have been brought to completion . . . without any intimation for the services of a physician who it is to be hoped has not merited this oversight." The offers of service on the part of his professional brethren, however honorable to them, wouldn't require very much work on their part, since, he asserted, very few patients would need serious surgical assistance.

The Duke's reply was placatory; he had probably discussed the matter with Whitbread: ". . . the offer does you credit . . . appointment of a physician essential . . . you should be that physician . . . the regulations you suggest will probably hereafter be adopted" and so on. But he agreed with Mr. Whitbread that if the plan for remuneration were to be put forward at that time, it would most probably fail.

That was enough to discourage Dr. Yeats. He abandoned his proposal and agreed to take the post of medical superintendent in an honorary capacity. His letter of acceptance, which consisted of only one sentence, was in marked contrast to those received by the magistrates from the surgeons, Charles Short and John Pulley [p. 19] and is worth quoting in full as an example of Yeats's personal style:

> "Gentlemen. The Lunatic Asylum for the County of Bedford having been brought to a degree of completion fit for the reception of a considerable number of lunatics whose diseases will require medical aid and it being moreover enacted in the 16th section of the 40th of the King, under the authority of which the asylum has been built in a situation which may afford a probability of the vicinity of constant medical assistance and it being further enacted in the 5th section of the 51st of the King, which is an amendment of the 40th, that the medical superintendent of every such asylum shall make regular returns of the persons committed to his care, that according to his report the Justices may dismiss such as are not fit objects to be relieved, it will give me much satisfaction gratuitously to discharge the professional duties of physician and medical superintendent to this institution.
>
> I have the honor to be, Sirs, G.D. Yeats"

* Author's italics.

Whitbread was in the chair at the meeting when that letter was read to the assembled magistrates and clearly, it required a reply of equal gravity. For this the committee turned to the Rev. Dr. Philip Hunt who had been chaplain to the Duke as Lord Lieutenant of Ireland (while Yeats had been his personal physician).

Hunt wrote that he was desired by the committee to thank Dr. Yeats for his very liberal offer; they had the utmost satisfaction in appointing him to discharge the important duties of that office. The committee was convinced that the appointment would strengthen the confidence of the county at large and that the friends of the unfortunate persons confined to the asylum would "derive hope and comfort from knowing that it thus affords every advantage which medical skill and science could supply towards the cure or alleviation of the most distressing calamity incident to human nature".

Philip Hunt had been appointed as one of the Bedford magistrates in 1811 and was closely connected with the management of the prison as well as with the affairs of the asylum. Born in 1772, he had graduated from Trinity College, Cambridge at the age of 16 and he became Rector of St. Peter's in Bedford in 1799.* Shortly after his arrival, however, he was given the post of chaplain to Lord Elgin, who had been appointed ambassador to Turkey. During the next six years he became an authority on the antiquities of Greece and was made responsible for removing the Elgin marbles and shipping them to England.

Stockdale† quotes Hunt who wrote of ". . . the destruction wrought daily by the janisseries of the fortress [the Parthenon]. They break off the finest bas-reliefs and sculptures in search of the morsels of lead that unite them to the building, after which they are broken with wanton barbarity".

On his way home overland, Philip Hunt was interned under a decree of Bonaparte's and it was not until 1805 that he was able to return home. But he hadn't been back for long before the invitation came for him to join the Duke (and Dr. Yeats) in Ireland. Stockdale says that he may have been chosen for his being of the Whig persuasion (as was the Duke), but also because Hunt was "a very

---

* County Record Office: CRT 180/166.

† In *Law and Order in Georgian Bedfordshire* – see Bibliography.

broadminded man in religious matters, who could not stand bigotry".

Although the asylum was declared "compleated and ready to receive lunatics and other insane persons" at that meeting in April 1812, that was not quite the case. John Wing reported that an extension of the sewer was necessary and it was ordered that it be prolonged "... through a close of the Duke of Bedford's occupied by John Coles into a spring by a gun-barrel drain of matching diameter".

There remained the question of the furniture, equipment and clothing. Samuel Whitbread had not been idle in this respect; he had consulted Thomas Dunston, the manager of St. Luke's Hospital, who had given evidence at the select committee hearings. Whitbread now read out a letter from Dunston, who was going to send (on the Bedford wagon) the following articles for use at the asylum:

1. A drawing of the iron railing round fireplaces "and it may be proper to add that a short poker is fixed to the stove by an iron chain".
2. A typical bedstead with a bolster, three blankets, a pair of sheets and a "coverlid . . . I have given directions for a bedstead on an improved plan which you may perhaps wish to have when completed, if not, I shall keep it for myself".
3. Two patterns of strait waistcoats, one for men, lined and of stronger materials, the other for women.
4. A pair of handcuffs, these to be of various sizes "and also the leg locks and to open with the same key".
5. A leg lock.
6. A chain for arm and leg locks to be fixed by a staple in the bedstead, wall or floor. "The length must depend . . . on circumstances and the nature of the case."
7. A pattern of a japanned iron chamberpot – "better than wood or earthenware".
8. Two tin mugs for beer, broth, gruel etc., the largest size for men, the smaller for women.
9. A pattern of trencher – "better than a square shape and not so liable to break".

If some of the items in that grim catalogue caused any qualms among the members of the committee, they went unrecorded. This was 1812, and it was not until the following year that Samuel Tuke's "Description of the Retreat, an institution near York" was published.

In 1791, a Quaker girl had died in suspicious circumstances a few weeks after her admission to the lunatic asylum in York. The Society of Friends, led by William Tuke, decided to create an institution:

> ". . . under their own care, in which a milder and more appropriate system of treatment than that usually practised might be adopted."

The first patients were admitted to the Retreat, as it had been named (to signify a place of repose), in 1796. It is generally agreed that Samuel Tuke's account of the institution came to exercise a profound effect on the way in which the mentally ill were treated, not only in this country but internationally.

Under the Tukes, the insane were accorded "the dignity and status of sick human beings". Their system was designed to replace the brutalities and methods of "restraint" in general use. The usual medical treatment was given a trial – bleeding, purgation etc., but failed to work. One remedy, immersion in a warm bath, was found to be useful in calming agitated patients. For these, too, it occurred to the superintendent to take a leaf out of the book of nature; animals in the natural condition tend to sleep after a meal. The provision of food to patients in a maniacal state helped to calm them and to give them (and others within earshot), similar relief.

The founders of the Retreat rejected the use of fear, i.e. threatening words and behaviour as a method of treatment. Attention was to be paid to the general comfort of the patients, and "no chains or corporal punishment are tolerated on any pretext in this establishment".

> "If it be true," wrote Tuke, "that oppression makes a wise man mad, is it to be supposed that stripes and insults and injuries, for which the receiver knows no cause, are calculated to make a madman wise?"

It was, however, conceded that violent patients ought to be segregated for their own and others' protection.

But, for the Bedford asylum, all that was for the future; the building was ready, the high walls were in place and the windows securely barred. A bell was still needed at the front gate and the governor, William Pither, was instructed to obtain flock stuffing for the beds from Mr. Trapp the draper. He was to obtain, from the same supplier, the materials for the patients' clothing – sufficient for 30 patients of each sex:

For each man; a coarse woollen jacket and trousers, three shirts, two pairs of stockings, shoes, a hat or cap, neck handkerchiefs and a night cap.

For women; a coarse woollen gown and two petticoats of the same material, two caps and one "bonnett", two pairs of stockings, three shifts, stays, three aprons and shoes.

As for the style of these garments, Pither was instructed to go and inspect similar articles at the county gaol and to find out from the gaoler where the clothing for the prisoners was made (probably the House of Industry, the town workhouse) and to follow suit.

The governor was also to procure a large-sized mangle, and some wooden spoons for the patients' use.

By July 15th 1812, George Allen had been appointed by the chairman, John Miller, to the post of keeper and his wife, Jane, to that of "keeperess", at an annual salary of 15 guineas each. Thomas Wiseman was to be the porter and his wife (also named Jane) the laundress, at 10 guineas each.

Advertisements had been placed in the *Northampton Mercury* during the previous month indicating that the asylum was now in a fit state to receive patients.

The Visiting Justices now addressed themselves to the task of tracking down suitable inmates and persuading the parish overseers to hand them over.

CHAPTER THREE

Making a start: Yeats v. Pither 1813-14

Preliminary enquiries by the parliamentary select committee had produced a nil return of lunatic paupers; it seemed that there were none in Bedfordshire. The survey which, according to Dr. Yeats, Whitbread had commissioned (and of which no record has been traced) had, however, suggested a figure of 147, and it was no doubt on that number that John Wing's original brief for an asylum of 100 places had been based.

In 1809, the magistrates, who reduced the figure of 40 on grounds of cost, had circulated the overseers with a demand for exact information about potential inmates living in their parishes. Now that the asylum was truly ready to receive them, only 12 applications had been received.

This was "... far below what it is supposed must be the real number of objects fit to be sent to the asylum from the different parishes in the county". Parish officers who had not responded to the previous circular were to be reminded of "the penalty to which they will be subject in cases of failure of their duty in neglecting to report paupers [who were] fit objects of the protection of this institution". In all cases where returns were made of "ideots [i.e. the mentally subnormal] or lunatics" who were not dangerous, the officers reporting them had to produce certificates to that effect from the parish medical officers.

The magistrates' clerk, Mr. Pearse,* was instructed to send out a new printed letter in rather more vigorous terms than the previous one. No doubt it also conveyed the information that the County Treasurer, Francis Green, had been appointed to manage the finances of the asylum, and that a weekly rate of 12 shillings was payable to him by the overseers for each patient sent in by them to

* Theed Pearse, a noted local solicitor, was Clerk of the Peace and Town Clerk from 1810-1816; he was succeeded in succession by his son and grandson.

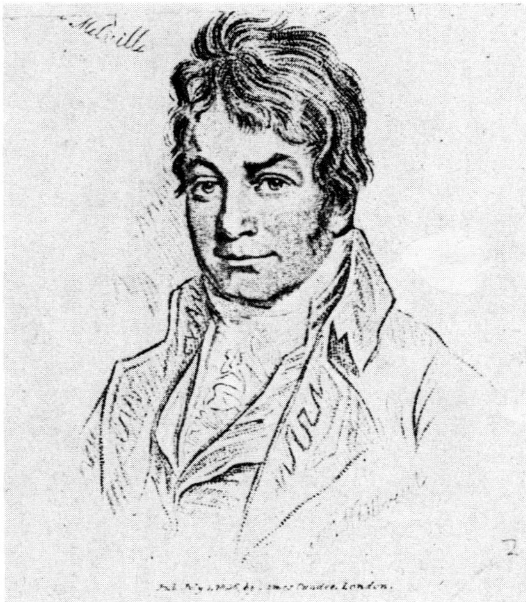

Samuel Whitbread –
print by Cundee c.1806. County Record Office

defray the cost of care and maintenance, medicine, clothing and the salaries of the officers and attendants.

The overseers were thus subjected to a dual financial squeeze; they would be fined if they didn't comply, and it would cost them if they did. The variety of their replies says as much, if not more, about the letter-writers themselves as about the state of pauper lunacy in Bedfordshire, as the following selection shows:

> "Stotfold August 10 1812:
> Sir I rite to inform you that we have no more Lunatics for our parish At present But if any thing of the kind shold happen in our parish we will be Sure to let you now immediately Sir I am very sorry that I did not Answer the first Letter for I am no scoler But Mr Webster inform me that we Sold have rote to you soner w'en ever we receve A Letter from you Again we will Answer it immediately.
> Robt.Oliver J.Hide Overseers"

"Maulden August 1812:
Sir, this is to a Quaint you that we have no Lunatic That is Maintained by our Parish
From your Obedient St.
Edwd.Dowdeswell Overseer"

"Upper Gravinhurst
Sir You Mentioned that the Justices were surprised at my not givin Notice to Mr.Pyther of the Lunatic Ideots in the Parish but I received no other letter than that dated 20 of July but we have neither in our paris.
I am your Hum Servt.
J.Mann Overseer of Uper Gravinhurst."

"Sir this is to inform you that wee have No Such person as lunatick or Dangerous Ideot In our parish Witness My Hand James Adams over Seer in the parish of Ridgmont."

"Everton 2th. *[sic]* of August.
Gentlemen
I have this day received your letter and I take the earliest opportunity to answer it, I ham verry sorry that I did not answer the other, we have not any such persons as you speak of belonging to Our Parrish and that made me think perhaps it was not necessary but for my fault I Humbley ask you Pardon and shall Esteem it as a great favour if you will be pleased to look over it.
I ham Sir your Obedient Servant Wm.Curtis
We have no People but what is right from anything of that kind."

"Copel July 9:
This is to Inform you the one person Menched in the Former Letr Will Not come hur Freinds dont Chuseit Nor the Parish Dont think Proper. From the parish of Copel So no Moore
Sir your umbel servant" [Unsigned]

"Tilbrook August 11 1812:
Sir, In reply to your enquiries concerning lunatics etc. – I have

to say (with much satisfaction to myself and the parish) that there is no person falling within the description of the printed letter, now living within our parish. . ."

"Stambridge
Sir the overseers of the said Hamlet Meane to send you a man that is something bering in mind he as being sent to Mrs.Burrows* London about 4 months but no better – therefore we mean to send him the later end of this week if convenant.
Yr Humble St Jos Eames Overseer"

Origin obscure:
"Sir We have a Woman By the Name of Jane Webster wich is at Mrs.Burrows at Oxten wich wee intend to send to the Silom at Bedford as soon as she can conveniently be Gott Down." [Unsigned]

"The parish of Little Staughton:
Sur I right thes liens in Ancer to your letter to Infourm you that thir is no persons With in our parish of that Discrepon Mentioned in your letter
I am your obedient servant Overseer to the poor."

The overseer of Westoning had evidently taken legal advice:
"Sir
I received your letter in consequence of wheather there was any Ideot or Insane person . . . but having none I thought there was no necessity of wrighting to Inform you concerning such Business but I have learnt since according to Act of Parliament that proper notice should be given to you therefore Gentlemen I hope you will Excuse me for not wrighting sooner to acquaint you therewith . . .
Francis Boston Overseer."

From James Lilburne (Samuel Whitbread's agent):
"I am desired by Mr.Whitbread and the other overseers of the parish of Southill† to inform you that they have two female

* E. J. Burrow and son were the proprietors of a private madhouse in Hoxton.
† This was yet another of Whitbread's offices.

> persons of the description to be admitted into the asylum." The women were in a private madhouse in London, possibly Hoxton, and the parish wanted to be sure that there was room at the asylum before being put to the expense of removing them to Bedford. The reply, from Pither, was prompt – he asked for them to be sent in "as soon as convently".

His friend and fellow magistrate, William Wilshere, wrote to Samuel Whitbread on August 5th:

> "I have received 2 letters from Mr. Pearse respecting a lunatic (or rather an idiot) in the parish of Holwell, Beds. – the man is named Charles Rendle about 35 years of age, has through life been very harmless & every day goes to work; if his earnings are not sufficient for his maintenance the parish make up the deficiency – such a man does not appear to me a fit object for your Asylum. . . ."

Wilshere added that if any further certificates to that effect were required, he would attend to it. But Whitbread was not to be diverted from his course. In September, Pither reported that 58 parishes had sent in replies stating that "there were not any objects within their respective parishes coming within the description of the Act".

Sixteen, including "Ampthill, Biggleswade and Shitlington" had said that they had some disordered or deficient persons but gave reasons why they were not suitable for the asylum. Seventeen admitted that they had suitable candidates in their parishes but gave various excuses for not having referred them.

The letters were handed over to Whitbread, who announced that he would visit all 33 parishes in person to see for himself whether there was any justification for their failure to comply with the law. His travels in the course of this undertaking included the village of Holwell and at the foot of Wilshere's letter about Rendle he scribbled a note: "Visited Sept. 27/1812 . . . a harmless idiot".

Meanwhile, preparation of the asylum to receive patients continued. A bell was hung in the passage and connected to pulls in the committee room and in the matron's quarters. Two rows of hat pegs were installed on each side of the fireplace in the former, and a large mangle was placed in the basement next to the laundry. Rails were to be fixed "for securing patients" in various sites such as "the knife place and the ash-hole".

John Wing was asked to "bevil the set-off of the wall . . . to prevent the patients getting over". He replied that raising the walls would, in his opinion, be more effective.

In July 1812, William Leech attended and accepted the part-time post of medical-attendant-in-ordinary at a salary of 20 guineas per annum.

Discussion then turned to the question of the various responsibilities in managing the institution. (Dr. Yeats was not finally to accept his unpaid post until four months later and wasn't invited to attend this meeting.)

The important matter of the patients' food was considered and it was decided that the ordinary diet would consist of:

Dinner (12.30 pm.): Meat on four days a week; on meat days, ¾ lb. of undressed meat with "a proper proportion" of bread and vegetables. On non-meat days, dinner consisted of broth "in which the meat of the previous day shall have been boiled".

Breakfast (8.30 am.): Oatmeal gruel and a small portion of butter with bread.

Supper (7.30 pm.): Bread and cheese.

Table beer was allowed at all meals.

The diet for any patient could be altered only on the advice of the medical officer, but it was the duty of the governor, William Pither, to regulate the hours of rest and airing of the patients. No visitors were to be allowed except by written order by a magistrate, but it was within the governor's powers to refuse to comply in such cases if in his opinion the visit was likely to harm the patient. Reasons for refusal were to be noted on the order for the magistrate to see.

Supplies were to be arranged on the same basis as at the Infirmary i.e. by local tender.

The cost of maintaining each patient was set at 12 shillings per week and it fell to the secretary, Leech, to calculate the amount of money due from the respective parishes, and in due course, to collect it. A record was to be kept of all persons visiting the asylum and of who authorised them to do so. Visiting hours were to be from

10 a.m. to 6 p.m. In this way, a visit from Samuel Whitbread with his family on the night of July 31st was duly noted.

By then only 17 patients had been admitted; according to Pither none were recovering except for a John Harper who "conducted himself very quietly and was particularly attentive to keep his clothing neat". The governor reported that, because some of the outer walls were too low one patient had escaped and another was on the point of doing so when he was observed. All the male patients had therefore to be kept locked up. John Wing was asked to give priority to raising the walls, and complied almost immediately. Nevertheless, Edward Hatton escaped on two occasions (but was recaptured each time).

The justices were firmly in control of the admission and discharge of patients – Whitbread insisted on the transfer of a sick patient, Rebecca Saunders, to the Infirmary, where his influence (even though it had not the same legal backing), was considerable. Alas, she died shortly after her admission there. At the meeting in September 1812, when only Samuel Whitbread and the Duke of Bedford were present, Leech (the house surgeon and secretary), reported that two patients, Elizabeth Fossey and Elizabeth Green, were both at that date "in enjoyment of a lucid interval".

There were then only 20 patients in residence, 12 male and 8 female.

The two women were called before the Board and were questioned: Elizabeth Green was found to be "perfectly sane" but declared herself "quite satisfied and pleased with the treatment that she had received and . . . interested to stay in for the time being". Her discharge was deferred. Elizabeth Fossey was "much amended in her mental health although not quite free from mental disease . . . she expressed great satisfaction in the care and treatment shewn to her and great aversion to being moved". She too was allowed to stay.

Dr. Yeats was appointed physician to the asylum in December 1812, a post in which he was Leech's superior. A month later he wrote to Whitbread:

"In looking over the inhabitants of the Lunatic Asylum there is one poor creature who requires more indulgence than I wish to take upon me to order. . . ." If Whitbread was going to Bedford on the following day [the letter was addressed to him at his home in Southill], would he be good enough to look in there and direct as he thought fit? A patient named Ann Kendal had been transferred from the Infirmary some time previously with "a deranged state of mind connected with the venereal disease", and he had found her rubbing in mercury in an attempt to obtain a cure. This, Yeats said, was dangerous; her cell, "though comfortable under normal circumstances" was too cold for a prolonged course of the treatment.*

There were still only 24 patients in the House despite Whitbread's exertions and as Green and Fossey were still willing to stay, they were retained.

Times were hard. The bills for December (for meat, bread, beer and clothing etc.) amounted to £130.10s.7d. and Leech was directed to request immediate payment of their dues from the parishes concerned.

It was resolved that up to 10 patients could be admitted provided that they were not paupers, that they had medical certificates to say that they were suitable and on the undertaking by "respectable housekeepers" [i.e. – holders] to pay 12 shillings a week for their maintenance – with the ordinary diet. Extra diet or other "indulgence" would attract additional payment. And so an element of private practice was introduced. With it came the opportunity to improve the finances of the asylum and to ensure fuller use of the facilities on offer.†

Friends of one of the existing inmates asked that he be provided with "better living". This was agreed, but only on condition that they paid 18s. per week on his behalf. The amount of bed linen was found to be inadequate and Mrs. Pulley, wife of the surgeon, presented sufficient material to make up 40 sheets (in the house).

The boot scrapers which had been ordered had not yet been fixed and Wing was informed that "the Board were dissatisfied with the delay and beg the job may be done". The keeper was allowed to shave patients upon an extra payment of one penny per head each time – but nobody more than twice a week.

---

* Mercury was in common use for the treatment of syphilis, which in its later stages could result in general paralysis of the insane, an illness which brought many of its victims into asylums. Yeats does not appear to have objected to the patient's treating herself, only to the temperature at which she was doing so!

† The nature of the problem, and the response, will no doubt be familiar to those concerned with such matters nearly 200 years later!

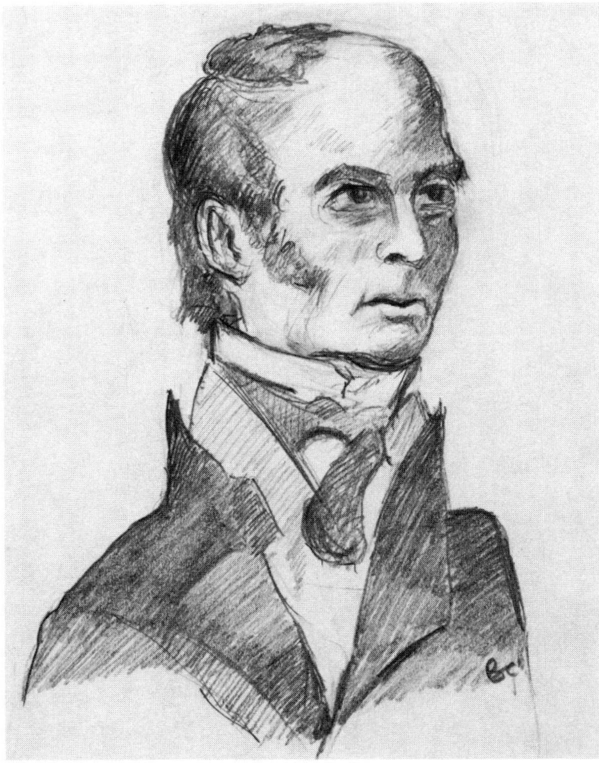

Drawing by the author from Garrard's portrait of Dr Yeats, c.1810

The extension to the sewer which had been agreed by the justices had been completed and now, to add to their worries, John Cole, the occupier of the land through which it passed alleged damage to his farm when the gun-barrel drain was installed. The claim was settled for £18.5s.0d.

"December 4th 1812: Thomas Fells an Idiotick Patient from Harlington died in the asylum . . . the cause assigned for his death is Hydrothorax, or water in the chest." He was buried at St. Mary's Church, where most inmates dying in the asylum were interred.

Early in 1813, Dr. Yeats began to busy himself in earnest with the affairs of the asylum. A battle for supremacy began between medical authority, represented by Yeats, and management, by the governor, William Pither. Which side was favoured by Whitbread is not clear. He had an interest in ensuring that the asylum was as fully occupied as possible, even if it meant keeping the Elizabeth Greens in for longer than was strictly necessary. For his part, Dr. Yeats was willing to discharge as many as possible, "to save expense to the parishes".

At the meeting on April 3rd, Whitbread was in the chair when the doctor brought a number of cases before the Board and several were duly sent home. But among the four who had been admitted was ". . . a female patient from Cardington where she was found wandering, dumb and unable to give an account of herself". It was suspected that her place of origin was in Eaton Socon, and enquiries were made of the overseers there – had a female pauper strayed, perchance, from their workhouse? The reply from the parish officers was immediate; they knew of nobody answering the description, they said.

Dr. Yeats submitted his first official report to the magistrates on April 21st. Characteristically, it was a document of eight closely written pages, beginning with quotations from the relevant Acts of Parliament and reminding the justices of their discretionary powers over all the measures to ensure the patients' recovery.

Apart from the need to make annual reports, he said, the functions and powers of the medical superintendent were not defined, and he strongly urged the adoption of regulations for "the separation of the different classes of lunatics from the convalescents" – clearly a medical responsibility. Many maniacs, he wrote, owned their disease to epilepsy, and he described "the condition of their countenances and the convulsed agitation of their limbs during an epileptic seizure, the intervals of which being filled up with loud and indecent vociferations".

Samuel Whitbread was probably well aware by this time of Dr. Yeats's tendency to generalise from the particular, and of his uncertainty in diagnosis,* an impression which must have been reinforced by the next request in the report. Yeats asked the magistrates to issue a notice requiring the overseers to obtain from the medical person providing the certificate of insanity a written statement "from his own knowledge" setting out the origin and *probable cause* of the condition. This, he asserted, would enable the asylum physician to apply his remedies with greater certainty! Then came the opening shot across the governor's bows:

---

* See *Private Charity and the Public Purse op. cit.*

> "The manager . . . of maniacs requires more than the usual strictness and obedience . . . I suggest the propriety of directing the governor of the servants [meaning Pither] implicitly to obey the physician in all things where the treatment of the patients is concerned."

This was followed by a broadside, clearly intended to disable his adversary. Employment of the patients was important:

> ". . . where any profit is desired from the labouring lunatics as in making lace . . . some proportion of that profit should be appropriated to themselves to keep alive the advantage of industry in their minds. None of the profit ought to go to any of the asylum servants – that would be an inducement to keep them at work longer than necessary." [Yeats proposed that a return be made to the justices of the profits from work done by patients.]

Although the report was addressed to the magistrates by Dr. Yeats, it was opened and read by William Pither, the "governor of the servants" to whom reference had been made, and he was greatly offended. His official designation on appointment had been plain "governor", as was that of the holder of the similar post at the prison and was comparable with that of "master" of the workhouse. Each had overall responsibility for those institutions, including for work done by the inmates.

Personalities apart, the episode was indicative of a much wider lack of general agreement about the definition of insanity, its varieties and causes, who should treat it and, of course, how.

On April 25th Pither sent a personal letter to Whitbread.* Although written in a meticulous copperplate, the spelling shows him to have been untutored, as Whitbread knew when he appointed him. But the strength of his feeling leaps from the paper: He was

> "Quight Struck With Astonishment" to know who had been talking to Mr. Whitbread, but on looking into Dr. Yeats's report – "I find he wass the Gentleman". Yeats had said that the

---

* Whitbread correspondence; W1/161.

servants should not have any benefit from the work of the patients. "Who wass Dr. Yeats calling servants – those in the kitchen?"

When Pither was in London, he said, he was a master tradesman ". . . and was informed by Samuel Whitbread Esq. that I was coming to Bedford to be Master of the Lunatic Asylum in my proper place". Yeats's remark that allowing the keepers any of the profit might induce them to keep the patients in longer than was necessary had evidently bitten deeply: "I Apele to you to know what opinion the overseers of the Diferant Parrishes Will have of me and what loss may be my own to have it Reported that I would for the Sake of a Poultery Bit of Lace . . . [confine anyone longer than was necessary.]"

He hoped and trusted that "our characters will not be done down by Dr. Yeats" and he didn't expect to be treated "like the Sum of the Earth when I was working in the garding with the patients".

No doubt he would be thought better of if he dressed himself up every day like a gentleman – he had always been upheld by work and hoped that he always would be, whatever his trade. If, as had been suggested, profits from the patients' work were to be given to them when they went home, then "everyone in the least bit sane would expect to make Lace".

It was for the magistrates, not the physician, to oversee his conduct, wrote Pither, but he ended his list of complaints by assuring Mr. Whitbread that he meant no disrespect to Dr. Yeats and that he wished to obey him in every respect as a medical gentleman.

Whitbread's reply was firm but diplomatic:

"I am extremely sorry that owing to my inadvertence the temptation was thrown in your way of reading the letter which you may have observed was addressed to the magistrates and ought not be have been read by you, but as you have read it, it is necessary for me to say that you have very much misunderstood the purports of that letter which certainly means to cast no reflection whatever on you or your wife but Doctor Yeats would not discharge the duty he has undertaken if he did not point out such circumstances as he thought deserving the consideration of the magistrates: and the matter relating to the lace I conceive to be so. . . .

"You will please to observe that these regulations are made not for you in your time nor for us in our time only; but for all future time . . . instead of considering it any degradation to you that you work with your men and thereby encourage them, I think it a matter of great praise to you that you do so. . . ."

The control by the physician was no more than was exercised at St. Luke's and at all hospitals of the same kind and it was absolutely necessary of course that it be attended to.

"I am," the letter concluded, "Your friend, Samuel Whitbread."

Shortly afterwards the justices resolved formally that "in all matters relating to the health and distribution of the patients with a view to their convalescence or their medical treatment" the governor was to obey implicitly the orders of the physician. It was further ordered that Pither was to render accounts relating to the manufacture and sale of lace and the sum of £3 was deducted from his bills for grass which he had sold without authority.

The matter ended there, with Yeats triumphant. In August of the same year, 1813, each of the protagonists had the opportunity of paying tribute in his own way to his referee. Writing to Whitbread, Pither thanked him effusively for a letter which we had received the previous day in which he had expressed "the satisfaction of the gentlemen magistrates with his work".

"August 11th 1913,* Dr. Yeats to Mr. Whitbread:
Dear Sir

Will you excuse me in requesting the favour that if you send or bring any gentleman of celebrity in attending maniacs to visit the Asylum, you will be so good as to allow me to accompany him as it would afford an opportunity of useful conversation – I mentioned to the Chief Baron† that your activity produced what he saw & of which he spoke in so much praise. His answer was that you are equal to any thing.

Dear Sir Yours very faithfully G D Yeats"

* County Record Office W1/165.

† The judges of the Court of Exchequer were usually barons. Patricia Bell suggests that this reference was possibly to Baron Parke of Ampthill.

In August 1813, it was noted that Pither had been engaged in work on behalf of the county from May of the previous year, although he hadn't actually arrived until June. He had not received any salary for a whole year – evidently it had been the intention to pay him 12 months in arrears. The magistrates conceded that this might lead to financial difficulties and resolved that Pither's salary would be backdated to May 1812 and that in future, the governor would be paid half-yearly.

Nevertheless, the magistrates were rigorous in their scrutiny of the financial state of the asylum; they had, after all, been entrusted with the handling of public money and the institution had to be seen to be paying its way.

Thomas Pindard, one of the patients, was to be discharged to the care of his parish officer. The overseer was told to remove Pindard that same day, and as the clothes in which he had arrived were in such a bad state that they had to be destroyed, "it was ordered that the parish do pay for the cloaths with which he was discharged".

Whitbread's suggestion concerning the supply of drugs and other items from the Infirmary had been adopted, and now resulted in a charge of £15.12s.6d. (for furniture) and of £51.15s.1d. (for drugs). The apothecary's bill for the drugs was to be examined and the friends and relations of the patients then in the asylum were to be required to pay for the medicines given to those patients.

Parishes in arrears were "to be written to . . . ordering immediate payment and that the same be enforced". (This threat was sometimes realised; in October, the parish of Bolnhurst was in arrears to the tune of £23.1s.6d. up to June 30th. Application was made to the court of Quarter Sessions to order "the proper process to compel payment thereof".)

The justices considered a payment of nine guineas to Dr. Yeats by Mrs. Slinn, a patient who was not a pauper, and in any case, not from Bedfordshire. It was decided that treatment of "out-county" patients was not part of the doctor's official (and gratuitously provided) duties and that if the patient's friends chose to place Mrs. Slinn under Yeats' care as a private patient, his proposed charges of one guinea on admission and half a guinea a week for the first six months were reasonable and "had the sanction of the Board".

Whether that sanction was enthusiastic is, however, doubtful. The means adopted by Dr. Yeats to enhance his private practice were in contrast to the circumstances surrounding the admission of the Rev. Isaac Hurst* as a private patient under the care of Charles Short, surgeon to the Infirmary and a prominent local citizen. Short had been mayor of Bedford on several occasions, and with his colleague John Pulley and others had engaged in a notorious professional dispute with Yeats in the case of Ann Fooks.†

A medical certificate from Charles Short had been produced at the time of Isaac Hurst's admission. His maintenance costs would be defrayed and it was directed "that he be treated by the keeper with all the attention due to his station compatibly with his mental health" – and with the asylum regulations. The patient had been under the care of the surgeon from the beginning of his illness and his friends wished him to remain so. The magistrates agreed to the condition.

Dr. Yeats decided to leave Bedford in 1814 and to try his luck in London; ". . . . to transplant myself to the metropolis and quit the early scenes of my professional exertions" was how he described the decision in his letter of resignation from the Infirmary. He continued to attend the asylum until his actual departure.

Dr. Joseph Thackeray's appointment to the Infirmary and his subsequent and distinguished career there is a matter of record.‡ After joining the hospital he wrote to the justices:

> "The obligations which the county of Bedford has been pleased to confer upon me by my late appointment of physician to the Infirmary entitles it to the service of my exertions in every matter in which its medical interests are concerned. . . . I trust that my utmost exertions to remove or alleviate the sufferings of the unfortunate beings it [the asylum] contains will gain me the only reward to which I look forward, the approbation of the magistrates who are its guardians."

The board instructed the secretary/house surgeon, William Leech, to return their best thanks to Dr. Thackeray for his offer of services "from which the patients would be materially benefitted".

---

* Probably the father of George Hurst and his brother Isaac, surgeon to the Infirmary in 1845 – see *Private Charity and the Public Purse.*

† *Ibid.*

‡ *Ibid.*

Ten days later, Leech (who was also secretary and house surgeon at the Infirmary) wrote a letter to Samuel Whitbread in which he complained that Thackerary had spoken sharply to him on finding that he had conducted a post-mortem examination on an asylum patient without the agreement of the relatives. Leech threatened to resign from the Infirmary because of the incident, but Yeats came to the rescue.

He wrote to Whitbread saying that Leech was unaware of Dr. Thackeray's appointment at the time of the row, and that all was now well between them. (Leech was, in fact, a key member of the Infirmary staff and must have been aware of Thackeray's appointment there on February 19th as well as of his letter to the justices quoted above.)

CHAPTER FOUR

Whitbread, Thackeray and others: 1814-27

It is doubtful whether Samuel Whitbread was in any state to lend much of an ear to such matters at this time. He was beset by financial worries connected with such enterprises as the rebuilding of the Drury Lane theatre, and much of his attention was engaged by national politics as well as by problems arising locally – at the Infirmary, the gaol, and in his magistracy. His connexion with the lunatic asylum had become well known and a number of letters to him on the subject have survived in his collected correspondence. For example:

December 13th 1813; from the Rev. E. D. H. Sexton of Chesham *[W1/5042]*

> "... To extend the influence of humanity in your public capacity as in private life I know is your pleasure. . . ." The writer had been a patient in a private asylum and deplored the ill-treatment that he had seen administered to his fellow sufferers. Weren't there regulations for houses of that kind? And was this a subject "worthy of cognizance of those who consult the internal welfare as well as the external defence of England?"

His close friend (also a leading Whig), Henry Gray Bennett, sent Whitbread a letter *[W1/5073]* from a Mr. Johnson full of complaints about the "inquisitorial power" enjoyed by the College of Physicians over private madhouses. And Edward Makepeice *[sic]*, writing from Lincoln's Inn *[W1/5075]* invited Whitbread to attend a meeting of the committee of "the London Asylum for the cure of the Insane" to receive a report of their sub-committee on the state of the insane in their places of confinement. There is no record, however, of whether Whitbread ever attended this or any other similar meetings.

The inhabitants of Tring, in Hertfordshire, were grateful to Whitbread, according to a solicitor, George Knibb, for his efforts to get one of their parishioners into St. Luke's. As some delay in her admission was expected, could he get the patient into Bedford?*

Lord Anson wrote to him in October 1814 for advice on the management of asylums, since he was interested in establishing one in Staffordshire and wanted it to be "as perfect as possible . . . I am convinced", he wrote, "that whatever you undertake must be well manag'd". He added for good measure that he had recently read Tuke's account of the York Retreat.

In December, Whitbread received from one H. Fraser a copy of a long letter [W1/5082] that the man had sent to the Earl of Glasgow. It began:

> "I am informed by one of my spies . . . that a man has been sent to Glasgow at your instance for the purpose of kidnapping my person and confining me once more in a madhouse." Cruel practices were sanctioned privately there, he wrote, "with the aid of well-fed and bribed physicians and surgeons who might condemn anyone who shall displease a noble Scots Earl, to everlasting misery in the dungeon of a madhouse – without trial, without judge, without jury . . .".

Fraser's ravings continued. He went about apparently alone, he said, but in reality was accompanied by 10 supporters who were ready to rush to his assistance. The letter concludes with a personal plea to Whitbread:

> "Having a high opinion of your goodness I forward you a true copy of a letter . . . I need not inform you [that] these measures make it your duty to bring the case before Parliament if you wish to save England from ruin."

During the early months of 1815, Whitbread's health declined, and his friends and colleagues were increasingly concerned. His speech is said to have become slow and slurred and he complained of

---

* Whitbread's link with St. Luke's Hospital was evidently quite widely known. William Smith, a fellow MP, sent on to him a letter from a man named Blackman alleging ill-treatment of patients – "atrocious barbarity" – there, including threats that Dunston would sell their bodies for dissection, and for "three or four pounds".

headaches and feelings of depression. Whitbread suspected that he was despised by everyone and unworthy to remain on earth.

On July 6th 1815, three weeks after Napoleon's defeat at the battle of Waterloo, Samuel Whitbread committed suicide at his London home. Five days later the Marquess of Tavistock addressed the House of Commons and described him as "the poor man's friend". Thousands of individuals had benefitted, he said, from his generosity and he had made "eloquent appeals in this House in favour of the unfortunate".

His memorial, and that of his father and other members of the family, is in St. Mary's church in Cardington.

After Whitbread's death, the asylum continued to expand, thanks to the efforts of, among others, Philip Hunt and Thomas Charles Higgins, of Turvey House. The latter became chairman of the Court of Quarter Sessions and continued as one of the visiting magistrates until the asylum closed in 1860. The justices received strong support from the physician, Dr. Joseph Thackeray, who reported to them every month on the state of the patients.

If his predecessor kept similar records, they have not survived, but by January 1816, there were 42 patients in the institution, 19 men and 23 women. Of these, 10 were private patients and the rest, paupers. Eight had been discharged during the previous month (and seven admitted). Sixteen of the patients had been inmates for four years i.e. since the asylum had opened.

In September 1815, Thackeray replied to a request which he had evidently received from Lord St. John to advise the committee on the functions of the medical department.*

In his letter Thackeray wanted to correct any impression that because only a few patients were receiving medical treatment at present, there was no need for such a department; the asylum was in its infancy and most of the patients were chronically disordered. In time, though, many more acutely ill patients would appear, needing "the active interference of Art".

He dissented from the generally held view that mental disorders were incurable, and argued that as physical conditions could influence the mind, it was reasonable to presume that "moral disorder" could be corrected by physical agents. Thackeray divided

* Dr. Thackeray's letter [CRO: LBP/1] is reproduced in full as Appendix 1.

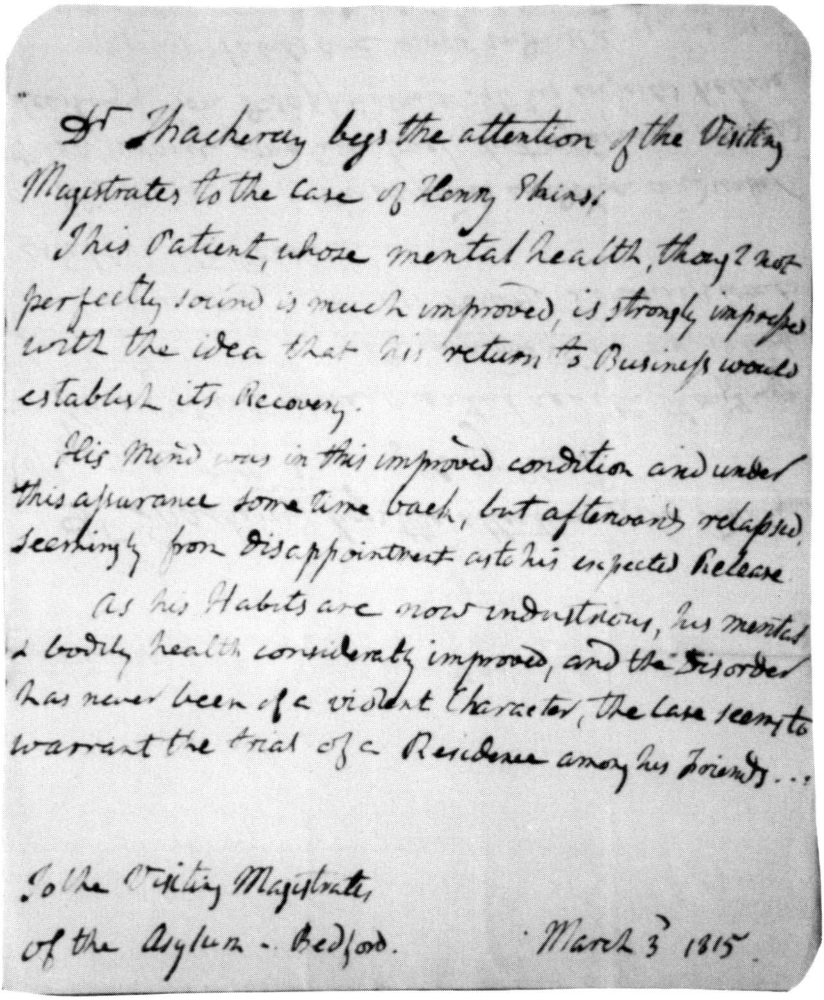

mental disease into three general classes, "maniacal and melancholic", both of which were connected, he maintained, with bodily disease, and "nervous", which was not.

Such a classification gave "great encouragement . . . for placing a lunatic asylum on the footing of a medical institution". But it would be difficult to get any suitable applicants for the suggested post of house-apothecary and secretary – the job hadn't the inducements to be found in, for example, a hospital. A salary of £50 (per annum) with board would be the least that could be offered "to a respectable young man", who should not be required to have a common table with the governor and matron.

When it came to recording diagnoses in the medical record book, Dr. Thackeray found it necessary to widen the field. In January 1816 for example, the largest group (12 patients) were labelled "insania", presumably the chronically mad. Among the others were:

Mania	8
Melancholia	10
Criminal lunatic	1
Amentia congenita	1
Insania epileptica	2
Melancholia religiosa	2

Dr. Thackeray's advice about individual patients usually demonstrated his humane attitude, which was to become increasingly evident at the Infirmary (where the problems were of course more overtly medical in nature). Psychiatry, as a medical specialty, was not to develop until later in the century and as his letter to Lord St. John shows, Thackeray's views reflected the maelstrom of an era in which the "new" science, the old poor laws and the rights of individuals were all under scrutiny. Roy Porter has produced a lively and detailed account of the various views of insanity* which prevailed at that time and some of which found expression at the Bedford asylum.

When recommending several patients for discharge in August 1815, Thackeray said that:

> "Alice Martin still continues weak in body and mind as this weakness seems now to be occasioned by separation from her children and as she is very steady in regard to the circumstances that led to her confinement, her release is proposed in the hope of its salutary effect upon her bodily and mental health."

Another, Mary Rumball, would in his opinion benefit from a return to the company of her friends. His recommendations for a dietary table were examined by the board and the governor was ordered to comply with them "as far as circumstances will allow".

---

* R. Porter, *Mind-Forg'd Manacles* – see Bibliography.

The justices were particularly attracted by the proposal that meat days be only three times a week and that the bread allowance for each patient should not exceed 14 ounces. After a trial period, Pither reported that there had been no difficulty (among the patients) with the diet table except that the discontinuation of small beer had produced much dissatisfaction. He was given permission to dispense it to such patients as he thought fit "unless prohibited by Dr. Thackeray in particular cases".

Samuel Whitbread's last attendance at the monthly meeting of the visiting justices was on January 7th 1815 (the Earl of Upper Ossory in the chair). Dr. Thackeray reported that Elizabeth Wildman was not insane but suffering from epilepsy "not of a severe character"; William Leech, the house surgeon, concurred. The magistrates decided that as she was "not a fit object for the asylum" the officers of her parish were to remove her forthwith. However, it emerged in the course of her examination that her father was at the time "confined in a private madhouse in Bethnal Green kept by Tarboys and at the expense of the parish . . .". The overseers were ordered, under pain of the statutory penalties, to apply to a magistrate for the father to be moved to the Bedford asylum.

In October 1815, Philip Hunt, no doubt prompted by Thackeray, arranged for a set of books to be obtained for the use of the magistrates, the medical superintendent, the resident apothecary (soon to be appointed in accordance with the doctor's suggestion) and the governor:

1. All the statutes relating to lunacy and "ideocy";
2. Highmoor's *Law of Ideocy and Lunacy*;
3. Reports from the Committee of the House of Commons concerning madhouses (private asylums) in England;
4. Tuke's description of the Retreat at York;
5. Haslam's observations on insanity and melancholy;
6. Dr. John Mason Cox's practical observations on insanity.

The medical report book was kept meticulously by Dr. Thackeray up to the time of his death in 1832. Prominent among the causes of death or discharge that he recorded were: hydrothorax (water on the chest), erysipelas, dysentery and apoplexy (usually in the aged). Epilepsy and dropsy were common and some simply died of "old age". Leonard Rainer, a pauper aged 71, succumbed to a gangrenous foot, and a melancholic female private patient from Biggleswade strangled herself with a neckerchief.

In 1818 Thomas Peck suffered so severe an attack of "inflammation of the bowels that he needed "more assiduous attention than could be given in the House". He was transferred to the Infirmary, where he was treated successfully, and after his return to the asylum two weeks later, the house surgeon there presented a bill for £7.12s.2d. in respect of the expense of the extra nurses required; the justices settled the account without demur.

It was sometimes necessary to choose between patients; John Allen, a pauper from Northants, who had been an inmate for five years, was removed to make a place for a Bedfordshire pauper. The design of the asylum was fairly inflexible, and in the 1820s the total number of patients during the decade remained at about 52, divided equally between men and women. On average, three patients were discharged and four admitted every three months.

The justices were fully aware of the possible risks to the patients and to the asylum's reputation when they returned patients to "the community". On January 7th 1822 Thackeray reported that because of overcrowding, it would be necessary to discharge one of the patients who had come from outside the county; he recommended the removal of Ephraim Wells of Ivinghoe, Buckinghamshire. The nature of the man's incurable malady, he said, rendered him very burdensome to the institution. The justices agreed and the patient was discharged.

Two weeks later, the Earl of Bridgwater wrote to the Bedford magistrates enclosing a letter from John Lloyd, a surgeon, who had been asked to examine Ephraim Wells at the workhouse in Ivinghoe:

> "I found him in the same state of alienation as before, and very weak. I examined his body carefully and found a great many bruises particularly his right knee which was much inflamed and an abscess has since formed. His legs, arms, back and head have contusions on them which appear to me to have been inflicted with some blunt instrument, they cannot I think ... be the effect of falls."

The surgeon's letter ended by saying that "the poor man speaks incoherently of being beat with a large stick and violently kicked", but that he was now clean and comfortable at the workhouse and was being treated with great humanity.

The governor, William Pither, was called before the justices and began by reminding them that they themselves had ordered Wells's discharge.

> "... I gave him into the care of his brother and of a young man who accompanied him. They took Ephraim Wells away in a one-horse cart at 8 o'clock in the morning; he could walk better than when he was admitted. During his stay in the House he frequently fell down ... and often bruised his head by such falls and once both his eyes were rendered black by a fall."

Pither said that the man "was very ideotic" and that great attention had been paid to him. He had been treated with the greatest care and *never* beaten – anyway, "none of the keepers had any sticks".

William Agutter, keeper, confirmed what the governor had said. "I can appeal to all the other patients to prove that Ephraim Wells was kindly treated by the officers and by the other patients." He had washed him from head to foot on the day of his discharge and found two bruises from previous falls, and he had also found "a boil on his knee which he had when he first came and which was not quite healed". When a convalescent patient said that he could confirm that "every care had been lavished on Ephraim Wells" the magistrates reached the unanimous opinion that Wells had been treated with the utmost care and tenderness while he was in the asylum.

In succeeding months, however, Dr. Thackeray was careful to draw the board's attention to any events in which the treatment of patients might be called into question. In May, he reported a serious accident which had occurred when a patient, Thomas Rabin, fell from a railing; the circumstances would, he said, be related by the governor. "As the effects of his fall required great care and nice surgical treatment, I took the liberty (as he was in a very calm state of mind and not likely to be troublesome) of having him removed to a private ward in the Infirmary, where he is now lying in a most dangerous state." The magistrates examined the railing and ordered its replacement. Thomas Rabin died six weeks after the fall.

Samuel Crouch had been admitted as a private patient on the application of his mother and two weeks later was found dead in his cell, suspended by his braces and handkerchief from the iron bars on the window. At the time of Crouch's admission, his wife had assured Pither that her husband was "perfectly harmless and not inclined to do himself injury if no particular temptation was put in his way". The governor reported that a coroner's inquest had "sat upon the body who returned a verdict of lunacy".

By 1822, the magistrates were becoming increasingly critical of William Pither's management of asylum affairs. He had been governor since Samuel Whitbread had appointed him when the institution had opened in 1812 and after the departure of Dr. Yeats and the arrival of Dr. Thackeray, was careful not to encroach on strictly medical territory.

When, in 1818, a farmer named Brown, who owned an adjoining field, had presented his bill for 17 shillings and sixpence in respect of three acres of grass ("an extraordinary charge") it transpired that the governor, anxious to have fodder for the asylum cows in the following winter, had purchased the crop and made it into hay with the assistance of some of the patients.

The justices had to approve the plan but made plain their objection to its having been effected without their prior approval by deferring payment of Pither's salary and incidental expenses "until a more numerous meeting". (Only two, Captain William Waldegrave* and the Rev. George Cardale, were present.)

In November 1822, Philip Hunt reported to his colleagues that on a visit to the asylum in September he had been greatly concerned to find that on ringing the outside bell, the door was opened by one William Bean, a criminal lunatic, who had been committed to the Court of Assize after killing his two children in a fit of insanity. On enquiry he had found that the governor was absent and that the under-keeper had not been put in charge of the keys. Pither admitted the facts but said that Bean's behaviour was so much

* Captain William Waldegrave, RN (1796-1838) was Samuel Whitbread's son-in-law, having married Elizabeth, the latter's eldest daughter. The two men were close political friends, and after Whitbread's suicide, Waldegrave was "hustled" into his seat in the House of Commons. He occupied it until William Henry Whitbread was old enough to take over and to represent Bedford in Parliament – from a personal communication to the author by Mr. Waldegrave.

improved that he had no hesitation in leaving him in charge. The justices delivered a severe admonition and:

> "... explained to the governor that patients who are committed to this asylum by order of the assize courts as criminal lunatics are to be considered as convicts sent for safe custody; and that they must be kept as securely as if in a prison; and with the same responsibility attaching to the governor."

William Bean died of "inflammation of the windpipe" in April 1823.

The visiting justices, as always, kept a close eye on the finances of the institution in general (and the governor's accounts in particular). They didn't shrink from applying pressure to defaulters – overseers of the parishes or those who had accepted responsibility for private patients. Mr. Osborne of Cranfield was in arrears of more than £20 in 1823 for the maintenance of a Mrs. Odell, aged 70, probably a close relative; it was "ordered that a premptory *[sic]* application be made to him ... unless the arrears be immediately paid, Mrs. Odell will be delivered over to him".

She had been admitted as a private patient a year earlier and Thackerary described her as suffering from "insania". Her bodily health was "good" but her mental health "bad".

(A similarly peremptory letter was sent to the overseers of Stanbridge on another matter; unless they paid up, a prosecution would immediately begin against them. It was later decided that three months' payment in advance would be required.)

Mr. Osborne was in trouble again the following year; in September he owed £23.18s.0d. for Sarah Odell's maintenance. If he failed to pay by November 3rd she would be sent to him and proceedings would be instituted to recover the debt. The deadline arrived and Osborne had paid £6.10s.0d. on account with a promise of £2 the next day and £7.3s.0d. at Christmas. But that would still leave the payment for three months in advance undischarged. He was informed that unless all the arrears were cleared before Christmas Day, Mrs. Odell would certainly be removed to Cranfield. A satisfactory conclusion seems to have been reached; she remained in the asylum until her death (from "haemorrhage") on April 26th 1826.

Nevertheless, justice was usually tempered with mercy. The

Duke of Bedford was in the chair in March 1822 when Philip Hunt produced a letter he had received from a Miss Dolbier saying that because of a reduction in her and her brother's income, she was unable to continue paying £1 a week for his maintenance.

An order was made that "in consequence of the diminished price of provisions and the increased value of the currency", the scale of fees generally would be revised. The new charges would be: pauper patients from Bedfordshire, 9/- per week; paupers from other counties 11/- per week, and private patients, 12/-. Miss Dolbier's fees were reduced.

The case of Sarah Peck: In June, the overseer of Great Staughton, Huntingdonshire, applied in person for Sarah Peck to be discharged (probably to save the cost to the parish of her maintenance), but the governor was of the opinion that she was unfit to go home because of the fears she had expressed that "she might destroy her children if she did so". When Sarah Peck was called before the committee, she repeated those fears and said that she had "temptations and bad thoughts" towards her children though she loved them dearly.

The magistrates agreed that it would be improper to discharge her, but as they had discovered in the course of their enquiry that her husband and the family were now living in Eaton Socon (Bedfordshire), decided that instead of moving her family back to Gt. Staughton, Sarah Peck would, *for maintenance purposes only*, be considered a Bedfordshire pauper.

This meant that the parish of Gt. Staughton would have to meet the lower fees – a saving of two shillings a week. Needless to say, the overseer was in complete agreement!

However, at the next meeting, the justices were informed that it was "now surmised" that the patient was in an advanced state of pregnancy and the matron, Mrs. Pither, caused some consternation when she gave her opinion that the birth was likely to take place within the next 10 weeks. It was therefore determined that Sarah Peck would be removed to her family "in a proper manner" as soon as circumstances allowed* and only if she was "in a state of mind as to render her removal justified".

* There were no facilities for maternity cases at the asylum or at the Infirmary. If she had not been able to go home, it might have been necessary to transfer her to the workhouse.

She was discharged home "on account of pregnancy" on July 26th.

On June 2nd 1823, Thomas Maclear, the surgeon, apothecary and secretary at the Infirmary (with similar duties at the asylum) submitted his resignation. John Harris, who had earlier been appointed to Maclear's post, was elected to fill the vacancy from September. He was destined to remain at the asylum, in posts of increasing seniority, until the institution closed in 1860 (when the Three Counties Hospital was founded at Arlesey).

An idea of the incidental expenses which had to be met may be gleaned from a fairly typical month's bills (January 1823):

Smith . . . Meat	£25. 9s. 3d.
Green . . . Grocer	£13. 5s. 3½d.
Whitworth . . . Butter	£ 2. 6s. 8d.
Langley . . . Draper	£30.10s. 5½d.
Trapp . . . Draper	£23. 3s. 3d.
Bunting . . . Draper	£19. 6s. 3d.
Hinde . . . Glazier	£10.15s. 1½d.
Wells . . . Baskets & clothes lines	£19. 6s. 3d.
Servants' wages	£21.16s.10d.
Master's incidents	£ 2.10s. 9½d.
Pulley . . . Draper	£ 18.18s. 7d.
Bunting . . . Carpets etc.	£ 8. 1s. 4d.
Total =	£180.13s. 2d.

Vegetables, milk and butter and beer were produced at the asylum, usually with the help of the male patients, while the women did the sewing and washing. It will be noted that nearly half of the above costs were taken up by four drapers, which may be explicable in the light of the following list of the annual requirements in October 1823:

"44 yds. of sheeting and shirting;
150 „ blue print;
125 of bed furniture;
125 coverlets;
24 prs. of blankets;

60 yds. of flannel;
20 „ brown holland;
70 „ Scotch sheeting;
200 „ calico;
40 „ linen ticks;
30 „ checks;
2 pieces of stuff for petticoats;
20 yds. of fustain *[fustian]*;
20 „ toweling;
12 „ of stuff for stays;
4 dozen of men's hose;
4 „ of women's ditto;
12 bonnets;
5 dozen neck-handkerchiefs;
2 „ pocket „ ;
12 yds. of muslin for caps;
50 „ of sheeting;
Tablecloths *[quantity not stated]*;
Tape, worsted, thread and cotton. Needles, pins etc.
Total estimated cost = £113.12s.0d."

In August 1823, the asylum received a visit from Thomas Dunston, the governor of St. Luke's Hospital, who had given practical help in setting up the institution. He "very much approved of the order of the establishment".

The records show that in November, the total number of patients was 56 made up of:

Bedfordshire paupers.................	male 19,	female 17	= 36
Paupers of other counties.........	male 1,	female 4	= 5
Private patients..........................	male 9,	female 6	= 15

The governor's salary in 1824 was £20 per quarter. A carpet "in imitation of the Brussels pattern" was ordered for his parlour by the justices – possibly indicating their recognition of the enhanced status which accompanied such relative affluence.

As always the magistrates were cautious about loss of revenue to the county. One way in which such loss might be sustained was if pauper patients were admitted without a legal order having been

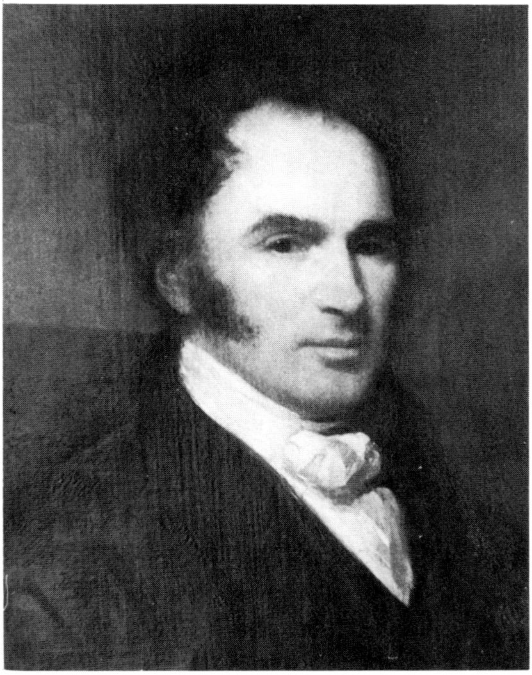

Detail of portrait of Dr. Joseph Thackeray by John Jackson, R.A. Photograph by Arthur Ferguson

made on the overseers to foot the bill. The governor was ordered to refuse admission without such a warrant.

Dr. Thackeray's request for a period of sick leave from his (honorary) duties was characteristic of the man. His health, he wrote, had been in a very indifferent state for some time and in compliance with the wishes of his friends he had decided to withdraw from his professional duties for a while. As giving a fortnight's notice would delay the opportunity to recruit his health, ". . . I venture to anticipate your indulgence and trust that I am not guilty of presumption in calculating to this extent upon your goodness". If the need arose, John Harris would be able to consult the surgeons to the asylum, John Pulley and Charles Short. (Thackeray was back in post 10 weeks later, his health much improved.)

A private patient, Elizabeth Squires, succeeded in getting hold of a knife and cutting her throat; Pither reported that "every practicable precaution had been used to prevent the melancholy occurrence".

"**William Hamilton,** a vagrant, his case":

In April 1825, this man, described as a vagrant lunatic, was apprehended in the village of Blunham and put in the charge of the parish constable by the minister and the overseer. They conducted him before Philip Hunt, who committed him to the Bedford asylum with a request that the medical superintendent and other officers do their best to find out where he had come from and to restore him to his family and friends.

William Hamilton was brought into the committee room, and the story that he gave would not have been out of place in a novel by Fielding or Smollett. It was detailed and free from inconsistencies:

> "He states himself to have been born at Bellingham in Northumberland where his father resided; that his father was afterwards a ship-owner at Greenock and lived in Dumbartonshire, that he himself was early entered in the East India Company's service, that he has been second mate of the William Pitt, East Indiaman of 1,400 tons, Cap^{n} Hope. That he lost £900 placed in the hands of Mr. *[name left blank – this was a serious charge!]* of Collingwood Street, Newcastle upon Tyne; that his brother is captain in the 13th Dragoons in the East Indies; that he himself had a bad typhus fever in Bengal [and], that he had been in the employ of Robinson and Hunter in Greenock."

Hamilton said that he had formerly been under the care of a Dr. Rawley at Lichfield, was known to the Dean and had been in the Hoxton asylum.

> ". . . he was once well taken care of by Mr. Cressy-Angel from Blyth near Nottingham who wrote to his friends and procured a guide to attend him to London and purchased clothes for him . . . he has of late been driven about by constables and robbed of a silver watch with his name engraved on it, and of money."

William Hamilton was discharged in September and was given £1 to defray his travelling expenses.

By 1825 the deficiencies of the building and grounds were becoming evident. In February, it appeared to Philip Hunt that "the cold generated in the lower cells (where patients unconscious and insensible to the calls of nature are confined) produce bad effects ... causing mortifications* and other dangerous maladies".

A Mr. Cutler, an engineer of Gt. Queen St., London, visited the asylum at the invitation of William Henry Whitbread and reported that the building "possessed every desirable facility for thoroughly warming the lower wards by means of two powerful air-stoves". The cost, including the wages and travelling expenses of the workmen, he thought, be about £80 to £85 for each – "the bricks and mortar and a labourer to be provided by the County of Bedford". Preparation would take six weeks and it would require a further eight weeks "to fit them up in a workmanlike manner".

The terms were accepted. It was then recommended that two more yards be added, one to each of the male and female sides "to enable such as are quiet and convalescent to enjoy air and exercise without being liable to be interrupted by the noise of frantic violence or immoderate mirth of their companions in confinement".

John Wing was asked to draw up plans and estimates, and two books were ordered, one by Tredgold and the other by Sylvester. Both were on the subject of the heating and ventilation of infirmaries and asylums. Philip Hunt evidently believed in the closest possible supervision of such projects. In June, he visited Bethlem Hospital in the company of the chairman of Quarter Sessions, Sir Robert Inglis, and the Hon. Captain William Waldegrave, a fellow magistrate.

They were particularly impressed by the ample space devoted at Bethlem to yards and gardens for "the use and recreation of the patients without which all endeavours to improve the mental health or recovery of the insane are almost hopeless". On their return to Bedford, they recommended a considerable increase in the size of the grounds already approved. The surveyor, Mr. Gardener, and Mr. Elger, the contractor, were asked to confer, but the new estimate was such as to get the matter deferred until or unless approval were given at the next quarter sessions.

At this point John Harris, house surgeon and secretary, announced that he, too, had been visiting other institutions. At the Bristol asylum he had observed mounds of earth raised in the yards so as to allow the patients "to see the prospects in the neigh-

* Probably frostbite or "trench foot".

bourhood and to be amused by observing the various processes of husbandry work, the passage of carriages, travellers etc.". This, he said, would be of great advantage to the patients in the recovery of their mental health. The justices were impressed by his suggestion and ordered similar mounds for the new yards. (Alas for progress – in November a patient named George Youill died of internal haemorrhage caused by the accidental fall of some earth on his body while he was working in the new yard.)

The committee also ordered, for the yards, "black-painted boards and bits of chalk or unburnt pipeclay by which the patients may be enabled to amuse themselves" and "a strong post with a swing horizontal moveable lever". How much amusement, and of what kind, the justices expected the latter, gallows-like, apparatus to afford is not quite clear!

James Diaper escaped by scaling a wall with the assistance of some other patients "at a moment when the eye of the keeper was not upon him" but the fugitive was quickly recaptured in the town.

Mr. Elger was contracted to carry out the new work in the grounds in the sum of £1,345 in addition to which, the cost of installing the stoves for heating was not to exceed £280.

Because of the position of the new men's privies, cesspools were impracticable. But Elger said that connecting them with the main sewer would cost only about £90 from which the expected cost of the cesspools, £30, could be deducted.

The new work was completed by May 1st 1826, but some alterations to the privies were needed "to prevent inconveniences which at present prevail". The arrangements for warming the cells were satisfactory and maintained an average temperature of 62° Fahrenheit. The two stoves consumed more coal than the old fireplaces in the day rooms (but those didn't heat anywhere else).

Expenditure on the necessities of the house showed, in November 1826, a considerable increase over the previous year allowing for the fact that the average number of patients was 52 and the number in the governor's household amounted to 17, including children. Pither was called in and was told that unless there was "a very material reduction" in the scale of the expenditure during the following three months, the committee could not continue him in their service.

It further transpired that the governor's mother-in-law was

resident in his household without authorisation; he was ordered to pay six shillings a week for her keep. Pither admitted that he also kept pigs, and was ordered to "discontinue such practice". The committee noted that the tea supplied cost *eight shillings a pound* – he was desired to cease such extravagance and to buy tea "of a very inferior price".

After three months, the justices were at first quite pleased to find that the cost of butcher's meat had been reduced by more than a quarter, and that of groceries by about 40%; but closer examination of the figures showed that a large proportion of the meat was left for the consumption of Pither's household and that "the reduction has been . . . all but entirely effected in the patients' food". He was left in no doubt that from now on, his activities were under the closest scrutiny.

His accounts were examined by the committee quarterly, and by June 1827 they were satisfied with the reduction that had taken place in expenditure without its having been effected by any means injurious to the patients.

1827; the case of Lucy Wardle: In February, the committee of visiting magistrates were confronted by a serious complaint by her brothers about the treatment received by Lucy Wardle, who had died in the asylum. It was said that her teeth had been broken, that she had been plunged into a cold bath as a punishment and that she had been left at night without a nurse when she was "in fever".

Dr. Thackeray and John Harris were asked to say what they knew of the matter. The justices also questioned the matron (Mrs. Pither), Mary Query, the keeper who had attended the patient and Elizabeth Woodland, a convalescent patient due to be discharged in the near future.

Having heard the (separate) statements, the magistrates "had great pleasure in recording their conviction that the report [had] originated in misconception". They were satisfied that the patient had had only one tooth, that she had extracted it herself and had presented it to the aforesaid Elizabeth Woodland.

John Harris had strongly supported Mrs. Pither, who, he said, always gave the best possible attention to the patients; he had no reason to think that Lucy Wardle had been ill-treated. Nevertheless, both he and Thackeray took the opportunity to stress the need for *resident* medical aid for the patients – a similar recommendation had been made in the visitors' journal by "the medical superintendent of the Bicêtre and another foreigner . . .". (Philippe Pinel was, in fact, renowned as a pioneer in "striking the chains off the inmates of the Bicêtre", and with Tuke and Chiarugi as one of the founders of psychiatry as a medical specialty.*)

The complaints were taken up by the Rev. G. Spencer on behalf of the brothers. In submitting the letter to the committee, Dr. Thackeray said that he was now satisfied that Lucy Wardle had not been ill-treated, but he remained worried by the possibility that she had been threatened by cold baths if she persisted in her refusal to take nourishment. He considered that the former "keeperess" ought to be re-examined, but the justices did not agree to take any further action.

In retrospect, it seems likely that the relatives were in the right; the practices involved in forcible feeding were denounced by John Haslam† in a letter to the editor of the *Literary Gazette* in 1821:

> "It is a painful experience to recur to the number of interesting females I have seen who, after having suffered the brutal operation of 'spouting' . . . have been restored to their friends without a front tooth in either jaw."

* Roy Porter, *Mind Forg'd Manacles* – see Bibliography.
† Dr. J. Haslam (1764-1844) was the apothecary at Bethlem Hospital until 1816.

CHAPTER FIVE

John Harris, surgeon and manager: 1827-31

By 1827, nine county asylums had been established in England:

Asylum	*Date*	*Approx: cost*	*Places*	*Initial cost £ [Per head]*
Nottingham	1811	£21,000	80	262
Bedford	1812	£10,000	52	192
Norfolk	1814	£35,000	102	343
Lancaster	1816	£60,000	170	353
Stafford	1818	£36,000	120	300
West Riding (at Wakefield)	1818	£55,000	250	220
Cornwall (at Bodmin)	1820	£15,000	102	147
Lincoln	1820	£12,000	50	240
Gloucester	1823	£44,000	120	367

Kathleen Jones* wrote that "since the staff of the average county asylum was so small it is hardly surprising that both keepers and doctors tended to rely on mechanical restraint as the one method of keeping patients quiet and orderly . . .". Furthermore, under the Act of 1808, keepers who allowed patients to escape were subject to fines which could amount to the equivalent of a month's wages.

Dr. Paul Slade, resident surgeon at Lancaster, described and illustrated a method of restraint of his own devising. It consisted of a leather muff with iron wrist locks. A more severe form had leather sleeves ending in single muffs and various chains, straps and leg locks.

The muffs were later added to the equipment at the disposal of the keepers at Bedford and with the manacles, chains etc. were in use for many years despite the doubts expressed by certain of the magistrates, such as T. C. Higgins and Henry Littledale. The arrival

* K. Jones, *A history of the mental health services – op. cit.*

of the Commissioners in Lunacy following the passage of the Lunatics Act of 1845 (as will be seen later) gave powerful support to the views of those who had absorbed the evidence coming from the York Retreat and elsewhere.

In 1827, a select committee of the House of Commons under the chairmanship of Robert Gordon, a Dorsetshire magistrate, produced a report which resulted in two Acts of Parliament. The first of these was applicable to private madhouses. The second, the County Asylums Act* of 1828 was, says Jones, "largely a measure of consolidation, but it provided in addition for a certain degree of centralisation".

At Bedford, the justices' copy of the Act bears signs of careful study, as did their subsequent actions. The visiting justices of asylums were now obliged to send annual returns of all admissions, discharges and deaths to the Secretary of State, Home Department, who had "the power to send any visitor he chose to inspect any asylum".

In the provinces, as at Bedford, two justices and a medical visitor were to be appointed at quarter sessions to visit four times a year and to report to the Home Department.

The Act did not give specific instructions about treatment, but did insist on regular medical attention. Establishments having more than 100 inmates (which the Bedford asylum did not) were to have a resident medical officer; those having fewer had to be visited by a medical practitioner not less than twice weekly. Restraint was now to be imposed only by order of a medical practitioner – a physician, surgeon or an apothecary.

February 4th 1828: The total number of inmates was 57.

Bedfordshire paupers:	(m.17,f.20)	=	57
Paupers from other counties:	(m. 4,f. 1)	=	5
Private patients:	(m. 9,f. 6)	=	15

The records of admissions and discharges which formed the basis of the annual reports, and which the justices now had to submit to central authority became more elaborate and included details of the

* 9 Geo.IV c.40.

occupation of individual patients – paupers and labourers and (presumably for the private patients), "lady" or "gentleman".

There were farmers (one of them described as "a criminal from Bedford gaol"), a wool-comber, a butler, a toll-keeper, a whitesmith and a collar-maker as well as soldiers, millers and shopkeepers.

The lists included at least one mad hatter. William Wright, aged 34, of Huntingdon was admitted on August 18th 1827 and, sadly, died two years later.*

The case of Isaac Birdsey: Some patients were admitted, or transferred from prisons, as criminal lunatics by order of the Secretary of State, Home Department. The overseers of Maulden applied for the release of one such, Isaac Birdsey, who had been committed after assaulting his mother. Dr. Thackeray reported that his conduct had been good and a Mr. Overman of that parish had promised to give him constant work. The justices agreed to his discharge provided only that the verdict of the jury at Birdsey's trial had been, simply, "guilty", and not "guilty on account of insanity" (in which case they had no authority to release him). His confinement continued, and the matter was not raised again until three months later, when John Harris reported that Birdsey appeared not to be insane but only ill-tempered.

In his opinion, this was liable to degenerate into mania if he were detained for much longer. The head keeper confirmed this view and said that Isaac Birdsey had spoken the previous night of his mother as "a damned old bitch". The man was called before the committee and questioned. He admitted to having used "that opprobrious term" but insisted that he had not been referring to his mother, although he declined to say who it was "lest it lead to consequences".

It was decided, possibly with a tongue in the judicial cheek, that the right course would be for the Maulden overseers to write to the Secretary of State asking for Birdsey's release. The effect of that advice must have been electric; even if Mr. Dowdeswell was no longer in office at Maulden [see p. 28], most parish officers would have been daunted by the prospect. So it proved, and it was the Clerk of the Peace, Theed Pearse junior, who sent off the request. A warrant for Birdsey's release was received shortly afterwards.

---

* The madness traditionally associated with this occupation has been ascribed to the inhalation of fumes of hot mercuric chloride used in the manufacture of felt.

By August 1828, William Pither, governor of the asylum for 16 years, had seen the writing on the wall. He informed the committee that a situation had presented itself for which he thought himself eligible, and that he wished to "consult the convenience of the Visiting Magistrates about the time of his departure". He offered to remain until October.

That suited the magistrates, who had been studying the new Act and were determined to implement it as far as possible. But first, they considered it prudent to restate their own position, in terms which would leave no room for doubt:

> "The major part of the Justices of the Peace acting in and for this County present, elected all the Justices of the Peace acting in and for this county to be the committee of Visiting Justices for the management of the lunatic asylum of and for this county."

The newly constituted committee now confirmed John Harris in the combined post of house surgeon and *manager* of the asylum.

His new salary was to be £200 p.a. "with board, fire and candle" plus "the further sum of five shillings a week for every private patient now or hereafter admitted into the House". Harris was allowed to take with him his pupil at the Infirmary, William Tuckwell, but it was emphasised that that was not to be considered a precedent; Tuckwell was not to act as a substitute for Harris, who would be charged £35 p.a. for his pupil's board.

Pither was ordered to prepare an inventory of all the furniture, linen and other articles belonging to the asylum, after which John Harris would check the list and take formal possession. The inventory itself throws further light on medical and domestic practice at that stage of the asylum's development, as the following extracts show:

"*Dispensary:*

A grate fixed; a green fender; a set of common fire irons;

A tank for water, with lead sink and pipe to carry off water with cupboard doors under, fixed;

A set of shelves, fixed;

A counter to fit in window with drawers &c; a writing desk;

A case for account books over;

A wooden stool;

A pewter ink stand;
A stomach pump;
A warm air lamp;
Cupping scarification lamp & glasses;
A pair of copper scales [and] a pair of brass do. in box;
2 sets of weights, 2 pewter measures, 2 pewter and one tin funnell, graduated glass measures; . . ."

[and, finally] . . .
"A lock on the door".

Sundry articles were kept locked up in the women's gallery:
"2 Bleeding pans; India rubber forcing bottle *[probably for forced feeding]*; 2 elastic pipes for do.;
A salve *[ointment]* knife and board; 4 pair of scissors;
3 salt cellars;
2 feeding boats;
6 bleeding towels; a medicine stand and bottles;
2 pairs of belts and gloves; 6 muffs and straps; 2 collars;
5 new strait waistcoats; 12 old ones;
12 wrist locks; 11 pair of police handcuffs;
3 pair of list shoes [and] 2 pair of leather shoes;
4 flannel bath bed gowns; 6 pails, brooms and brushes in use;
A chamber lamp for the sick."

In the men's new gallery (and not, apparently, under lock and key):
"A tailors shop board; a sleeve board; a goose; a shoemaker's hammer and hobbing iron; basketmaker's tools (12 of different kinds);
A set of straps for the bath; 5 pairs of hobbles or confinements for the feet; 2 collars; 7 pair of hand cuffs; 7 wrist locks; 3 leg locks; 4 pair of belts and gloves, 4 pair of straps; a long chain;
An iron hook for bed bottoms; a fire shovel, an oil can, 2 ladders, 2 dust pans [and] 3 shoe brushes."

The committee room contained one or two unexpected items:
"A pair of handsome moreen window curtains with french polished cornice &c. complete; a pair of white holland sun blinds complete; 9 Morrocco leather bottom mahogany

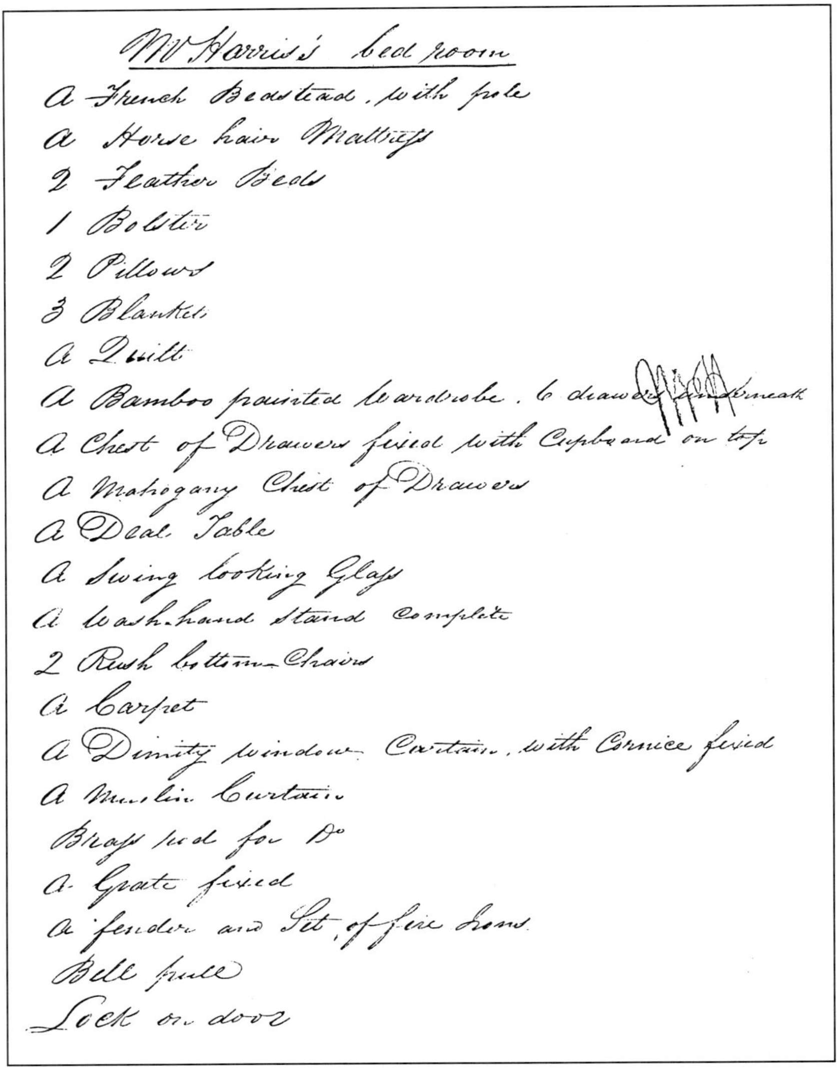

Mr Harris's bed room

A French Bedstead, with pole
A Horse hair Mattress
2 Feather Beds
1 Bolster
2 Pillows
3 Blankets
A Quilt
A Bamboo painted wardrobe, 6 drawers underneath
A Chest of Drawers fixed with Cupboard on top
A Mahogany Chest of Drawers
A Deal Table
A Swing looking Glass
A Wash-hand Stand complete
2 Rush bottom Chairs
A Carpet
A Dimity window Curtain, with Cornice fixed
A Muslin Curtain
Brass rod for Do
A Grate fixed
A fender and Set of fire Irons
Bell pull
Lock on door

chairs; a large table and green baize cover; a drab druggett to fit the room; an umbrella and hat stand; two small flower stands;

A barrel organ;

A head (study for phrenologists); 2 composition busts . . .".

Other items mentioned in the inventory included a bell pull, finger plates and a mortice lock on the door.

The first meeting of the new committee took place at the Shire Hall on October 14th 1828. Those attending included:

Sir Robert Harry Inglis, Bart. (Woburn) – chairman
Thomas Potter Macqueen Esq. (Ridgmont)
William Henry Whitbread Esq. (Southill)
Frances Pym Esq. (Hasells Hall)
Stephen Thornton Esq. (Moggerhanger)
Rev. Dr. Philip Hunt (Rector of St. Peter's Church)
Rev. George Cardle (Millbrook)
Rev. James Reed (Eversholt)
Rev. Thomas Barber (Houghton Conquest)

Thomas Narraway was appointed head keeper at £20 p.a. and, after a two weeks' trial, Mrs. Miles became the housekeeper at a similar salary. It was laid down that "no male be ever permitted to visit the female wards without the presence of the housekeeper". Two male and two female keepers plus a porter were still to be appointed.

Regulations for the general management were adopted and the committee was to meet monthly, as before.

Pauper patients were to be admitted at a cost to their parishes of nine shillings a week, but no private patient was to be charged less than a guinea. However, existing private patients would not be charged at the new rate retrospectively.

William Pither and his family departed with three months' salary, in addition to the arrears owed to him. The justices also allowed him £5 for about 60 fruit trees which he said he had planted on the premises.

It was ordered that the new general manager be allowed "to keep such a number of pigs as the offal of the house will supply with litter and food, and solely for the profit of the institution".

A chaplain, the Rev. H. Tatham, had been appointed and Harris (who had been asked for his observations on the improvements that were now needed) reported that the services had been well-attended. However, he considered that it would be advisable to place a screen between the male and female worshippers.

In February 1829, Harris visited two famous London hospitals "to learn about useful practices". At St. Luke's he was impressed by "the wire blinds to stop patients breaking windows by leaning on them carelessly", and by "a more simple and comfortable method of restraint than the strait waistcoat" (possibly leather muffs). He was attracted by the use of warm baths at Bethlem hospital and the "*entertaining books of history** and travel for the perusal of the patients".

On March 2nd 1829, John Harris submitted, at the request of the justices, his general views on the treatment of mental illness, while acknowledging that he had, as yet, no great expertise in the subject.†

Harris favoured a balanced approach between remedies applied to the body and those ("moral agents") directed to the mind – "I do not think that our attention should be exclusively devoted to the one or the other".

He recommended, for the able-bodied, activity of a kind similar to the patients' former occupations; farm work or in various trades. (He did not, however, venture to suggest any specific activities for the women.) In advocating the undoubted virtues of occupational treatment, Harris sometimes ventures into purplish prose: he aims to:

> ". . . break the train of diseased imagination . . . call back erring reason to her healthy course," rather than allow ". . . a confirmed madman to drag out a wretched life until death shall terminate his sufferings."

Nevertheless, practical suggestions were not lacking and the justices hired an extra eight acres of land for pasturage of cows, and acquired a hand-organ together with a number of improving books for the patients. At his suggestion, spouts were installed under the eaves to catch the rainwater for washing ". . . a great expense being regularly incurred for soft soap to soften well water".

The asylum was lacking in one serious respect – there were no facilities for warm (or even cold) baths, a deficiency which was noted by Dr. John Warburton, physician to St. Luke's, when he visited in 1831. They would, he said, not only increase the patients' comfort but would "in many cases materially assist in alleviating the disease under which they labour". Other visitors made similar comments but it was not until 1834 that warm baths and showers were installed.

When the family of Elizabeth Saberton wanted her to have a

---

* Author's italics.

† His report is reproduced in full as Appendix II.

separate room and the exclusive services of a female servant, Harris gave up his own bedroom for her use, and supplied the attendant. But the gesture was not entirely altruistic – it was agreed that the family would pay £2.7s.0d. per week of which £1.12s.0d. would go to the asylum fund and the rest to Harris.

He may have had other reasons for agreeing to give up his own quarters – there was a nasty smell from the kitchen and drains underneath his room, and the furniture was in poor condition. The committee agreed to pay Mr. Woodruffe the sum of £5 to remedy the inconvenience.

When Jane Stocks wrote to the justices complaining that she had been in service to the institution for 18 years (i.e. ever since it had opened) without any pay, Harris was asked to investigate. He was able to calm the collective conscience by assuring the committee that she had in fact been a patient, not a servant, for most of that time. Ms. Stocks was given £5 and told that her services were no longer required – somebody else would be engaged in her place.

The new manager of the asylum found that administrative duties occupied most of his time. When, as happened quite frequently, parishes fell into arrears it was John Harris who applied in person to the court of petty sessions for payment, and management of staff problems were his responsibility.

In 1830, Thomas Narraway, the head keeper, "had unfortunately acquired a habit of intoxication" and Harris recommended his dismissal. The man was called before the committee and "having heard the charge against him and answering it only by his tears" was told he would be discharged as soon as a successor could be found. (He departed, but was taken on again some 18 months later – as a porter at wages of seven shillings a week. It had been about twice that before.)

At the court of quarter sessions on January 18th 1830, Narraway's dismissal was confirmed and the justices agreed that a man and his wife should be appointed keeper and housekeeper in the place of "the parties one of whom is discharged by their order and the other represented as less fit than a married woman would be for her station".* Mr. and Mrs. Salmon were appointed head keeper and

* Twelve years later, riots at the House of Industry were to produce a similar recommendation from the magistrates – see *Private Charity and the Public Purse*, p. 20 – *op. cit.*

housekeeper respectively on November 1st 1830. Their joint salary was £40 p.a. plus travelling expenses from London.

One of the keepers, Samuel Fuller, applied for an increase in his wages of eight shillings a week; he found it difficult to maintain his family on so little. The medical superintendent supported his appeal; Fuller was, he said, "an excellent servant, most humane to the patients and most trustworthy".

It was evidently a test case. The justices granted Fuller an increase of two shillings a week, whereupon John Harris requested that a similar concession be made to Thomas Irons, another of the keepers, also on eight shillings a week and similarly excellent, humane etc. If the justices had any regrets at having risked bursting the floodgates, they went unrecorded and Irons, too, got his rise.

That they were by no means carefree in their disposal of public funds, however, was demonstrated when they received a bill for expenses incurred by John Odell, honorary surgeon to the asylum, in attending inquests on patients who had died there. While recognising the fact that they themselves had ordered that inquests be held on all such patients, the attendance of the surgeon was evidently considered part of his duties.

If the coroner wanted medical evidence other than that supplied by Harris (who would not receive a fee), they said, he would no doubt ask "some other medical gentleman in whom he had confidence".

It then appeared that Mr. Harris had the right to charge fees for inquests held at the asylum, but had declined to accept the money, for which he was commended, but the justices wouldn't accept his offer to give up that right, as they hadn't made a specific order against it.

The case of William Moseley: In November 1829: William Moseley of Huntingdonshire was admitted as a private patient on the warrant of Samuel Charles Whitbread and the Rev. Philip Hunt. He had been detained by the wish of his father's family but not it seems, that of his wife, who had been refused permission to visit him.

In July of the following year, L. A. Loudham, "Secretary of Lunatics to the Lord Chancellor" sent to "the governor or superintendent" a copy of a letter addressed to his lordship by Mrs. Moseley:

> "... I am a native of New York in the USA married to an English gentleman [who] has been confined in the lunatic asylum at Bedford for nearly twelve months past by the order of his brothers." John Harris had refused her request to visit him, she wrote. She attended the asylum daily but was given no explanation for the refusal. Mrs. Moseley asserted that her husband had lucid intervals lasting for weeks at a time and that she had approached the Board but was told that they "couldn't interfere with private patients".
>
> She had not wanted to take up too much of his lordship's time but she "... could if permitted relate almost unheard of cruelties as regards their taking him from me". Mrs. Moseley's letter ended with a plea for an enquiry or an order allowing her a weekly visit ... "grant the prayer of a helpless foreigner and your humble petitioner will as duty bound ever pray".

In September, the patient was brought before the committee. The Marquess of Tavistock was in the chair and Fred Polhill, MP, Philip Hunt and three others were present. Moseley appeared to them to be enjoying "an interval of perfect sanity" and said that he didn't want his wife to visit him. There were, he said, "circumstances connected with her conduct that would render any visit from his wife painful to him". John Harris concurred in the opinion that a visit from his wife "would be injurious to Mr. Moseley's state of mind".

The visiting justices confirmed the prohibition, copies of the relevant minutes were sent to the Lord Chancellor via his secretary of lunatics, and it had been demonstrated that it was possible for complaints about individual patients – private ones at any rate – to be taken up at the very highest level.

That ought to have ended the matter, but there is a brief postscript; on October 19th 1830, John Harris reported that William Moseley was sometimes subject to violence of such a character as to render him unfit to be continued in the asylum "with the present number of keepers". The authority to discharge him to the care of the family was granted.

At the same meeting, Harris took the opportunity (which may have been relevant in this case) to inform the justices that a number of patients had been admitted from other counties who were more strictly in the class of private patients and that some of the private patients "had descended to the scale of a pauper".

He proposed that patients from other counties, at present being treated by him "without profit" should pay more than at the existing rates. This was agreed and John Harris was henceforth to be allowed a proportion of the maintenance charges for all out-county patients, whether pauper or private.

The accounts for the financial year ending April 4th 1831 showed a total expenditure of £1,955.3s.3d., a reduction of £45 over the previous year. But Harris suggested that further savings could be made if coal were to be supplied on contract. Two tenders were received, each for the same amount; both offered "the best Blythe and Duck coal at 34/6 a chauldron, money". In a decision worthy of Solomon, it was agreed that Mr. Green and Mr. Barnard would each supply an equal proportion of the coal for the asylum.

Joseph Anderson and the blood horse: William Townrow, one of the Luton overseers, and Francis Field, a constable, produced a letter signed by two magistrates – Messrs. G. and M. Musgrave.

Joseph Anderson, a patient of the asylum, had been seen by Field and others "riding on a blood horse [a thoroughbred] in the town of Bedford and at other times breaking in colts instead of being confined in the asylum (if a lunatic) . . .". The Musgraves had happened to mention it to the visiting magistrates, who now summoned the witnesses who had observed Anderson at large to appear before them.

Francis Field stated that "on or about December 13th, he had seen Joseph Anderson, a pauper patient from Luton, riding in Bedford on a spirited horse, apparently a blood horse" – but knew nothing about his breaking-in any colt "or colts" since being admitted to the asylum.

John Harris was called in and said that he had never "granted to Anderson any liberty beyond what he thought necessary towards keeping him tranquil and contented".

As the patient had formerly been a gentleman's coachman and used to the management of horses, Harris had employed him to clean and exercise his own horse. However, he believed that the man was a confirmed lunatic, and that if he were in a situation where he could obtain intoxicating liquor he would probably relapse into violent mania. He declined, respectfully, to recommend Anderson's discharge [thus pleading, successfully, clinical freedom].

Another attempt was made to deprive John Harris of the services of his honorary groom three months later, but alas, Anderson was "not so well in his mind as he had been, and certainly not fit for discharge . . .".

CHAPTER SIX

A modest expansion: 1831-45

By 1831, the asylum was a well-established feature of the Bedford scene. A description at the time* called it:

> "a large and handsome building" standing at "a short distance beyond the Infirmary; having a beautiful shrubbery in front with a broad, semi-circular carriageway to the outer or wall-gate. . . . The entrance is handsome and the facade of the building might be considered light and beautiful but for the upper segments of the blank and arched windows, which alone are open; and which being furnished with iron bars, present the revolting idea of confinement . . .".

A few years later, Charles Allen, the treasurer of Middlesex, where a county asylum was to be built, asked a series of questions about the expense involved in financing the institution at Bedford (which had been, of course, a pioneer in such matters). The reply, by Theed Pearse, Clerk of the Peace, included the following observations:

(i) The expense of building and completing the asylum amounted to several years' ordinary County rates.
(ii) "The money was not borrowed on mortgage of the general County rates. A contract was made to erect the building for the sum of £9,585 to be paid as the work advanced by instalments of £550 at every Quarter Session until the whole should be paid . . . out of the general county rates which were to that extent increased and not by special rates."
(iii) There were considerable extra expenses in addition to the cost of the fabric, since six acres of ground were purchased as well as the cost of warming and ventilating the building and of the

* See Lynn Cater; *Beds. Mag.* XI, p. 58.

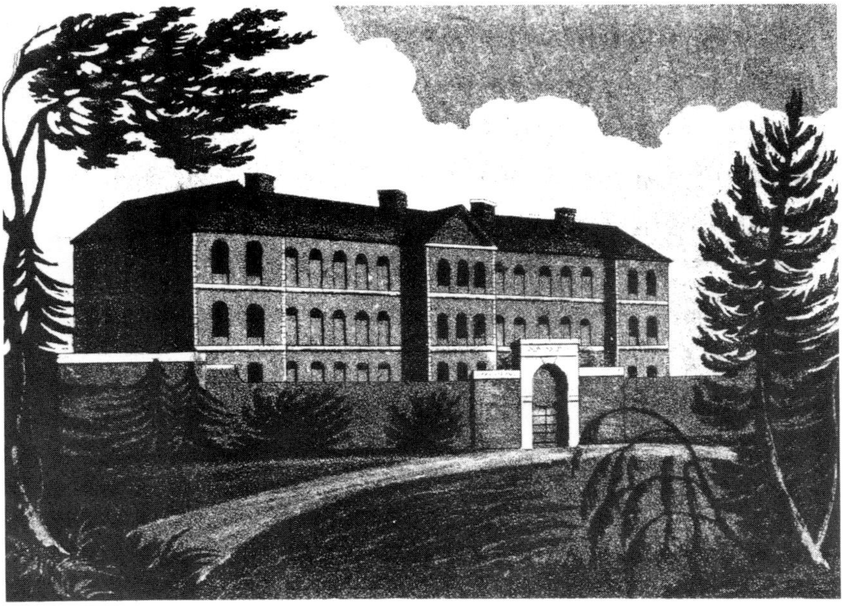

R.Hawell Junr. Sc. J.H.M.Del.

Lunatic Asylum.

patients' clothing. These additional costs amounted to £8,400 and were similarly paid by instalments out of the general County rates, as was the case with repairs and other expenses.

In October 1836, the total number of patients was 82:

Bedfordshire paupers	m.17	f.13	= 30
Out-county paupers	m.17	f.14	= 31
Private patients	m.12	f. 9	= 21

The expenses for the last quarter of 1836 amounted to £637.14s. 5d.,
this being met by payments from private patients – £255.13s. 0d.;
– out-county paupers at 9/- a week – £222.18s. 4d.;
– Bedfordshire paupers at 7/- a week – £137.17s. 6d.;
(plus balance in hand) – £ 21.17s. 0d.
Total balance – £ 2.12s. 0d.

When Harris asked the overseers of Biggleswade to remove William Barber, his nephew and another friend had written to ask that he stay, as they would have to find another institution for him. His income was "good", they said, but he would spend a quarter's rent in a few days and then starve for the rest of the time. They had no wish to benefit from his confinement and if he was allowed to stay, the whole of his income would be made over to the asylum. It was decided that subject to the usual conditions, he could stay as a private patient at not less than 17/6d. a week.

In 1828, an Act of Parliament* amended the laws for the erection and regulation of county asylums. Justices were allowed to appoint a committee of visiting justices to superintend the construction of the asylum and to manage it. That was already the case at Bedford. Similarly, there was nothing new in the permission to levy a county rate for the necessary expenses.

Another provision of the Act permitted the justices to borrow money on mortgage of the rates if they became burdensome to the contributors, but it was not found necessary to invoke this concession (which would no doubt be welcomed by the community charge or rate-payers of the present day). The Secretary of State for the Home Department was now empowered to employ any medical or other person to inspect and enquire into the state of any county asylum and report to him. Such inspectors were to be paid a fee for their efforts (by the asylum, of course).

Until 1828, the book in which visitors made comments was little used, but now the arrangements and the management of the inmates came under much closer scrutiny. There is no record of any inspection of the Bedford asylum under the terms of the Act of 1828, but the justices may have forestalled any such by drawing up a rota among themselves.

Prominent among them was Thomas Charles Higgins of Turvey House. He had qualified as a justice of the peace in 1821 and was elected chairman of Quarter Sessions in 1847. He retained that position until his death at Leamington in 1865.†

---

* 9 Geo.IV c.40.

† Obituary: *Bedfordshire Times*; February 13th 1865.

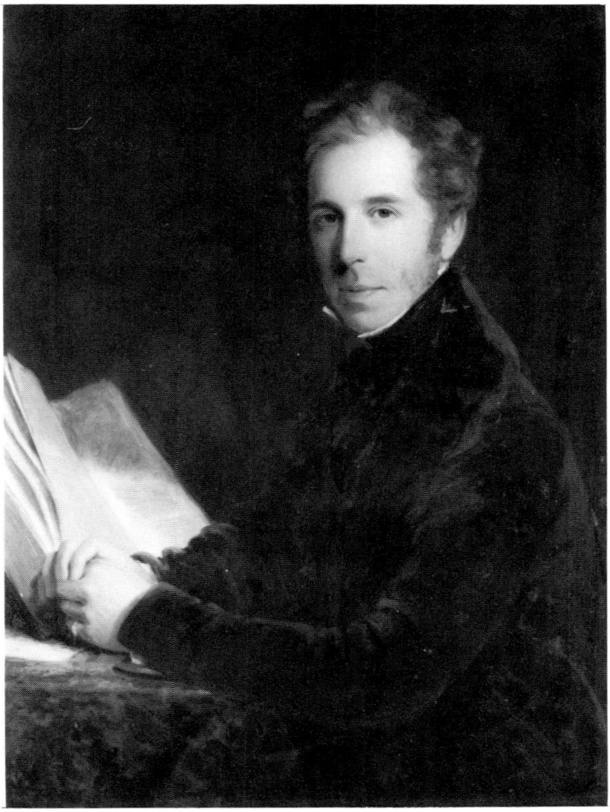

Thomas Charles Higgins (1797-1865) by W. Say.
By kind permission of Lady Hanbury

Throughout his career, Higgins retained a close interest in asylum affairs and it is not too fanciful to regard him as Whitbread's successor in this respect. His was the last official entry in the visitors' book when the institution closed in 1860.

The first of his observations was made on September 14th 1836; while the management was, he considered, excellent, he found some "most disturbing and appalling objects"; one man, for example:

> ". . . notwithstanding the most attention to prevent it, has accomplished his object in tearing off part of his tongue."

Higgins referred to Harris's intention to move out to his residence at a private asylum which he had established in Kempston.

". . . the more I reflect, the more certain I am that an asylum

> above every other institution requires the most assiduous, skilful and conscientious superintendent. The patients here are unable to communicate their sufferings and their wants . . . anything like negligence, indifference or harsh treatment will be much opposed to the present system."

Higgins believed that if the building were suitable, the asylum would stand pre-eminent, and considered that

> "however much wages should be allowed to the domestics by the justices as would ensure the most respectable class . . . much, after all, must depend upon those who minister hourly to the patients." The existing female servants were in his opinion too young and not sufficiently matronly. The language of the patients was frequently too disgusting and demoralising for such very young women.

On July 2nd 1832, Dr. Joseph Thackeray died, one of the first European victims of the outbreak of Asian cholera which had just made its presence felt in this country. He had earned a leading place in the affections of the people of Bedfordshire, not least through his work among the sick poor at the Infirmary,* and his death was the occasion of great public mourning. Thackeray's memorial, which was designed by Edward Blore, architect to William IV, stands outside St. Peter's church near the statue of another, more widely known citizen – John Bunyan.

By then, John Harris was firmly established in his position as resident medical superintendent and manager of the asylum, and the justices made no move to appoint another honorary physician to replace Dr. Thackeray.

For some time, Harris had been considering the advantages of opening a private asylum in the district and on June 30th 1835, he wrote to the visiting justices.

He proposed that:

> "in conformity with the recommendations of the France Committee, the present management of the lunatic asylum be altered and that it be confined entirely to an establishment for pauper lunatics. . . . In consideration of the reduction that would

* See *Private Charity and the Public Purse – op. cit.*

> consequently be made in his salary Mr. Harris proposed to establish a lunatic asylum for private patients on his own account, but to continue the medical superintendance and management of the County Lunatic Asylum at a salary of £140 per annum [reduced from £200] including medicines."

This was agreed and was to take effect from the following midsummer. Springfield Asylum opened in Kempston in April 1836 and the private patients then in the county asylum were transferred there shortly afterwards.*

In June, John Harris asked for permission to occupy the garden on his own account – either rent-free with vegetables supplied gratis to the asylum or at an agreed rental and be paid for the produce. It was agreed that he would take over the management of the garden, bear the whole expense of the same and provide all the vegetables required, free, in return for an allowance of £25 per annum.

The salary of the head keeper, Mr. Salmon, and his wife (the matron) was increased from £60 to £100 in recognition of their increased responsibilities now that John Harris had acquired divided loyalties, but there is little doubt that they resented their loss of income from the garden (the work in which was done by the patients).

A few months after the new arrangements had been implemented Salmon proposed that he take charge of the garden at the asylum and undertook to supply "all the vegetables required at no greater expense than £4 per annum for which Mr. Harris now receives £25". The justices agreed and furthermore ordered that:

> ". . . the patients in the County Lunatic Asylum be not in future allowed to go out and work at Mr. Harris's private establishment."

The asylum was not the only source of cheap labour; the looms at the workhouse [the Bedford Union] produced cloth which was used for bedding and for the clothing of the prisoners in the county gaol.†

A further example of reciprocity among local institutions

---

* Nigel Lutt's account of the establishment and subsequent progress of John Harris's private asylum is included here as Appendix III.

† Some years later, the Commissioners were concerned to find the female patients at the asylum dressed in ticking – a striped material used for mattress covers.

appeared when a baker named Pither offered "to take flour from the treadmills in the prisons and to make it into bread in a workmanlike manner and to bring it to the asylum at the rate of 3/9 a sack". But such an arrangement would, the justices decided, require them to give general notice that they wanted to change the existing system. Two months later the proposal to take bread using flour from the treadmills went out to tender. The lowest was from Geo. Clifton of St. Peter's (2/10 a sack). One month later Clifton lost the contract because of the poor quality of his produce and Thos. Bithrey, who had supplied bread in the past, was taken on, his being the next lowest tender. Pither, who had made the original offer, was not mentioned.

In 1836 the Hertfordshire magistrates appointed a liaison committee in order to consider more formal arrangements for sending their pauper and criminal lunatics to the Bedford asylum; a similar committee was being set up in Buckinghamshire for the same purpose. The Bedford representatives included Francis Pym, W. H. Whitbread, T. C. Higgins, Charles Longuet Higgins and George Peter Livius. After discussions had taken place, it was agreed that the Bedford asylum would accept criminal and pauper lunatics from Hertford (and from the "Liberty of St. Albans") for one year in the first instance.

Hertfordshire was charged at a weekly rate fixed according to the actual expense of maintenance and divided among the parishes concerned *pro rata* as at Bedford. This worked out at one shilling and sixpence per week for rent of the facilities, and seven shillings for maintenance of each patient.

The scheme was perhaps too successful; the asylum soon became overcrowded and in February 1837, Bedford was unable to accept more than 20 patients from Herts. When Huntingdon followed in September, the decision had already been made to enlarge the asylum and a special committee headed by Francis Pym looked to obtain a further 72 beds and enlargement of the asylum by about two thirds.

But that would cost in the region of £700, according to the architect, Francis Giles, who set out the specifications in a letter dated May 12th 1837*:

* [Footnote: CRO: LBP/7].

"My Lords and Gentlemen –
I beg to send you the particulars of the works suggested by you at your last meeting to be done in altering the lunatic asylum at Bedford as follows:

No. 1: To form on the eastern side of the building a sleeping ward for infirm or invalid patients:
A sleeping ward for unclean patients;
Day room; washing room; keeper's room;

Taking down the partitions – taking up the stone floor and relaying and providing as much new as will be required also a channel stone and drain to carry off the water; new doorways as shewn. Make good and limewash.

The whole of these will cost .... £ 37.10s. 0d.

No. 2: Build new day rooms; complete stone floor; timber roof covered with glazed sashes. New day room to cost .... £160.18s. 0d.

No. 3: Two new sleeping wards to cost .... £ 23.12s. 0d.

Total £222. 0s. 0d.

The like cost to be added for similar alterations on the western side of the building."

The existing accommodation of the asylum consisted of 80 beds and 1,050 [square] feet of dayroom space.

"The bedrooms can be increased for accommodating 72 additional patients and the day rooms can be increased to about 1,830 feet area making nearly double the present accommodation and extent of day rooms for the sum of about £700 which together with the sum necessary for additional warming to the building may amount to about £1,000, but as I have herein stated the alterations of the eastern end of the building may be made for £222 and those of the western end for the further sum of £222 exclusive of the warming.

Francis Giles."

Dr. John Warburton, MD, physician to St. Luke's Hospital, had visited the Bedford asylum in 1831, and while he was very pleased with "the extreme cleanliness . . . and the comforts that the patients enjoy", went on to recommend the provision of warm baths. They would, he noted in the visitors' book, not only increase the patients' comfort, but would "in many cases materially assist in alleviating the disease under which they labour".

In 1833, John Lee, one of the visiting magistrates, commented again on the absence of hot, or even of cold baths at the asylum. They were in his view "... considered almost essential to buildings of this nature". But he was very impressed by a plan of the asylum drawn up by one of the patients; it was worthy in his opinion of "being lithographed and a copy presented to every magistrate in the county".

It had been noted that Mr. Giles had neglected to furnish an estimate for warming the asylum. Mr. Elger was therefore requested to draw up the specifications "... as the season advances it is essential that some plan be adopted". Mr. Barwell* was asked to give his estimate for warming the two new wings of the asylum by warm water and "also to state what he will allow for the old iron per lb.".

(It was agreed that when two persons submitted identical tenders, the name of the successful one should be chosen by drawing lots, e.g. – "Samuel Lovell – Malt at 58/- per quarter for five months Poole and Hulatt – Ditto. Lovell is accepted.")

Two years later, Robert Inglis drew attention once more to the problem; the absence of baths was, he said, "a deficiency little creditable to us". He also suggested the provision of some means of opening the windows in the bedrooms – to facilitate through ventilation.

Proposals for other improvements to the building were put forward by various visitors; William Wilshere, a Hertfordshire magistrate and a close friend of the late Samuel Whitbread, suggested that for rooms which were going to be altered to accommodate "dirty" patients, floors of half-inch thick slate would be preferable to stone, being "cheaper, equally durable and not absorbent of moisture".

In 1837 the committee received from Barwell an offer to install apparatus for warming the asylum at his own expense "and not to receive anything for it till the justices are satisfied ...". If and when they were, the cost would be about £50. A tour of the establishment was undertaken in the light of all the proposals but the committee decided against recommending "these expensive alterations at the

* Possibly Edward Berrill, who submitted the ultimately successful tender.

TO

BUILDERS, Bricklayers,

AND

CARPENTERS.

THE Visitors of the *Bedford Lunatic Asylum* having resolved upon several ALTERATIONS and NEW WORKS therein, Persons desirous of contracting for the execution of such Works, are informed that Plans and Specifications of the same may be seen, and further Information obtained, at the *Clerk of the Peace's Office*, in *Potter Street, St. Mary's, Bedford*, where Proposals, sealed up, are to be delivered on or before the 2d Day of *June* next.

THEED PEARSE,
Clerk of the Peace.

BEDFORD, 26*th May*, 1837.

WEBB, PRINTER, BEDFORD.

present time". They noted that:

> "The county asylum at Northampton will shortly be opening and as it is proposed to receive patients there at a lower sum than in this county is considered practicable, it is likely that the number of patients in the Bedford asylum will shortly be reduced."

At the meeting in May it appeared that as the asylum contained 16 patients from Northants and that most of these would go to the Northampton asylum when it opened, the existing accommodation was adequate. However, the committee "ventured to recommend" that the day rooms be enlarged and the refractory cells altered as John Harris had suggested and that the plan for warming be accepted.

A poster was circulated inviting tenders for the work and a number of replies were received:

Richard Hands, for example, agreed to do the alterations in the men's and women's galleries "according to plans nos. 1 & 2: men's side for £42 and the women's for £45.10s.0d. [total = £87.10s.0d.]. He added: "PS my Tender of 75 Pounds is wrong Having Omitted some part of the Work."

Edward Berrill made a special offer, and although his arithmetic cannot have impressed the justices, it was his tender that was accepted:

> "Tender for work about to be done at Bedford County Lunatic Asylum
> Gentlemen
> I will agree to execute the work according to Plans & Specifications of East and West Wards each for the sum of Twenty Five Pounds Nine Shillings or Fifty one Pounds the two.
> Edward Berrill"

On July 3rd 1838 the justices ordered that a new dayroom be built on the men's side according to a plan previously submitted by Mr. Elger. The cost was not to exceed £150. Contracts were to be invited by advertisements in the press. The lowest tender was that of Geo. William Francis, for £200.15s.8d., and this was finally accepted on condition that he pledged himself to finish the work by the following spring. It was also resolved that Mr. Elger be requested "to instruct those patients who are bricklayers to make necessary alterations for making a new furnace mouth for heating the hot water".

A curious incident occurred early in 1839. Thomas Charles Higgins drew the attention of the court to an anonymous paragraph in the *Northampton Herald* of December 1st 1838. It concerned an accident which was said to have occurred at the Bedford asylum, caused by the bursting of one of the hot water pipes in the apparatus which had been installed by Berrill [of Northampton]. *No such accident had in fact happened,* Mr. Higgins told his colleagues.

But a few days afterwards such an incident *did* occur – "under circumstances of considerable suspicion". Clearly, an investigation was required. The Clerk of the Peace was instructed to write to the editor demanding the name and address of the person who had furnished the information – evidently someone possessing clairvoyant powers or else had contrived the incident. If any reply was received, the matter does not appear to have been pursued.

The old iron from the flues [which had been replaced] was to be sold "as well as the old small beer pipes".

"In consequence of repeated instances of broken windows" it was ordered that "part of some of the windows be bricked up and the remainder guarded by wire work." A tin blower was purchased to prevent smoke, and "if it do succeed a cowl be bought for the chimney; and use the old iron for guards to the windows".

Such precautions did not, however, prevent the Rev. Mr. Brown, a private patient, from throwing himself out of the window of the committee room on to the flagstones beneath. Fortunately, he "received scarcely any injury".

By 1839 the Bedford asylum was housing patients from Bedfordshire (40) and Bedford town (3); Hertfordshire (36); Huntingdonshire (12); Cambridgeshire (6); Buckinghamshire (4); Northamptonshire (2).

The justices were running short of accommodation not only for the living but also for the dead – the churchyard of St. Mary's, in which parish the asylum was situated, was overflowing.*

An order of court was made to set aside a piece of land to be consecrated as a burial ground for that parish.

April 28th 1838: From the secretary to the Bishop of Ely (John Burder):

> "The Bishop desires me to acquaint you that as far as his lordship is concerned he will readily and willingly consecrate the piece of

* See *Private Charity and the Public Purse*, p. 129.

ground in question but [some] bishops have declined to consecrate ground appropriated for the burial of persons dying in the Union Houses." This was, the Bishop had said, "in case the workhouse should be demolished and built elsewhere and the burial ground thereby become deconsecrated".*

If the ground were to be conveyed to the parish and treated as an extra cemetery, ". . . all difficulty would be removed. The Bishop does not throw out this hint to impede the measure but thinks it right to mention it".

A final paragraph mentioned the expense of consecration and suggested that the justices refer to the Registrar in Cambridge, a Mr. Twiss. The latter considered that the rule concerning workhouses should also apply to asylums, and once more referred them back to the bishop.

June 4th 1838: The Bishop of Ely finally agreed to consecrate a piece of land – "3 rood, 28 pole belonging to the county on the SE side of the asylum" for use as a burial ground.

The spiritual welfare of the patients was not neglected. The Rev. Henry Tatham, chaplain to the asylum, attended to his duties with great dedication and went so far as to submit his quarterly report to the justices in 1842 in the form of a letter written from "On board the *Dante* in the Straits of Messina". He was currently on a mission to Egypt and the Holy Land, he explained, and the Rev. Mr. Andrew would look after the spiritual interests of the patients until his return, ". . . if I am preserved to do so".

Henry Tatham was born in Buckinghamshire on December 18th 1788 and was appointed Rector of St. Cuthbert's with the strong support of the Duke of Bedford in 1822. After his travels to Egypt and Palestine where he made a number of important discoveries including a collection of Syriac manuscripts which aroused widespread interest in archaeological circles,† Tatham became Archdeacon of Bedford, an office whose duties he continued to perform after he was appointed Rector of Stanford Rivers in Essex in

* Prophetic words. The asylum was demolished in 1860 and the cemetery has disappeared.

† County Record Office; reference CRT 180/121.

1849. He received his Doctorate of Divinity from the hands of the Archbishop of Canterbury, was made FRS and received other honours, including his appointment as Chaplain in Ordinary to the Queen.

His obituarist says of him that "as a preacher he was not attractive, his elocution being kept so strictly in check as materially to mar the effect of many a good discourse". Nevertheless, Sunday services in the asylum chapel usually attracted a congregation of about 100.

D. C. Cooper wrote that he had visited the men's ward just as they were retiring for the night and was gratified to find that great quietness prevailed and that "one man was kneeling apparently very devoutly with his prayer book or testament before him".

On October 19th 1846 Henry Tatham reported to the justices:

> ". . . I know there is a widespread and deep conviction that it is utterly useless to attempt to carry the blessings which religion brings to the poor pitiable inmates of a lunatic asylum, as they are not in a fit state to receive them. But this is an erroneous conclusion, arising from a want of knowledge of the diversity of cases among the insane . . . I may refer to an individual who became a decidedly religious character in consequence of being brought to the asylum." (The man was said to have recovered but was readmitted some years later and eventually died in the asylum.)
>
> "In one of my visits . . . I happened to go into one of the dayrooms in the midst of an animated discussion, in which three or four were speakers and others sitting round the table listening to it with much attention." The chaplain asked what they were doing and one of them said: "We have been arguing about clergymen and ministers going to balls and plays and such places." At their invitation, Mr. Tatham joined the discussion and concluded: ". . . the many pithy observations advanced would not have disgraced a more sane assembly!"

Mr. Salmon and his wife, the head keeper and matron respectively, had been appointed in November 1830, and their salary was increased from £60 to £100 p.a. because of the increased responsibilities (when John Harris had opened his private asylum seven years later).

In September 1839, some discrepancies appeared in the household accounts and Salmon admitted to having indulged in what might, in the present day, have been described as "creative accountancy". A committee, consisting of Messrs. C. G. Payne, Samuel Charles Whitbread and Charles Longuet Higgins was appointed to examine the books, after which Salmon and his wife were directed to leave the asylum immediately. It was agreed, however, that while the accounts were under investigation, they would be provided with lodging and their expenses paid.

The posts were advertised and subsequently the justices resolved to recommend Daniel Porter of the Ampthill Union House and his wife. It is not clear whether that appointment was taken up but on June 1st 1840, Harris reported that the conduct of the incumbent, now a Mr. Thomas, was very unsatisfactory "in many respects". Thomas was given the opportunity to speak in his own defence, but the magistrates decided unanimously that he was unfit for the position and he was discharged with a month's salary in lieu of notice.

After a month or two's temporary tenure, William Pither and his wife Mary were re-appointed head keeper and matron. (They had left the asylum in October 1828 after having been there for 16 years, and had then been succeeded by Mr. and Mrs. Salmon.) Perhaps mindful of some previous problems, Pither's accounts were to be presented at each monthly meeting of the committee of visiting justices.

The accounts were to be ". . . kept in the manner of a Banker's book. A book has been provided in order that they [the justices, presumably] may always know the exact state of receipts and payments".

By December 1839 there were 118 patients in the asylum. This was too many and six months later Harris reported that as the previous Court of Quarter Sessions had recommended a reduction in the number of patients, there were 17 or 18 who were "quite harmless and inoffensive but not likely to recover". It would be desirable, he said, to report to the various Unions [of parishes] to get them removed from the asylum to those workhouses. The justices agreed. On October 7th 1840, Thomas Charles Higgins paid:

"an unexpected visit at the asylum . . . and took a minute survey over every part of the House; nothing could be cleaner, in better order or patients more quiet. Mr. Harris was there: I do not remember seeing the institution under such favorable circumstances and I regret the more that it does not afford such comforts and accommodation as the patients require in the furtherance of their cure and to which the present Head Keeper [Pither] would do so much credit."

Nevertheless, patients still escaped from time to time, Edward Coleman of Totternhoe had absconded while working in the garden, and Harris, in addition to informing the parish officers, was ordered to "request the Chief Constable of Police that search may be made throughout the county".

The recapture of such patients had, of course, to be paid for; bringing back John Williams in 1843 cost £6.5s.0d. and a failed attempt to locate William Stone (alias Barford) resulted in the expenditure of £2.8s.9d.

In that year, the property tax (the rates) for the asylum amounted to £1.12s.11d., and the justices paid West & Co. seven shillings for snuff. Claridge's bill for tobacco amounted to £1.15s.11d., in addition to which Willsher received five shillings and sixpence for mending scuttles and Bowes and Hester six shillings for chimney sweeping. Clayton charged a consistent 14 shillings for a coffin, but his other fees, for carpentry, were closely scrutinised; on one occasion, he had to appear before the justices to explain certain of these costs in person – evidently to their satisfaction.

When a patient died in the asylum, an inquest [sometimes referred to as an "inquisition"] was invariably held by the coroner, with a jury. In most instances, death appeared to be due to natural causes and then the jury brought in a verdict of "Died by the Visitation of God".

In other cases the verdict was more precise; at an inquest into the death of James Clarke the jurors found:

> ". . . that he died from the effect of pressure of blood and water on the brain and the death of the said James Clarke was accelerated in consequence of blows inflicted by John Saville" [a fellow patient].

No private patients were admitted to the Bedford asylum after Harris opened Springfield House and funding became even tighter.

In 1840, it was ordered that the maintenance charges for patients from other counties should be paid three months in advance, the amount being calculated from the previous quarter's charges. This provision was extended to all the patients in 1841.

When a Mrs. Kidman of Margate left a legacy of £500 for the benefit of the institution, the sum of £50 was deducted for legacy duty. The justices decided to provide a board recording Mrs. Kidman's and other legacies which was to be "stuck up in some conspicuous part of the House".

Despite all efforts to contain the overcrowding of the accommodation at the asylum, the numbers continued to mount. By 1842 there were 129 patients and in the following year the figure had risen to 136.

Similar problems had presented themselves at both the Bedford Infirmary, the voluntary hospital maintained by private charity, and at the Bedford Union, funded, as was the asylum itself, out of the rates.

The Infirmary had its Board of Governors and the workhouse its Board of Guardians. In the face of these financial and logistical difficulties, justices, governors and guardians all reached the same conclusions; the strictest economy would have to be exercised in the use of the available resources (although they didn't express it in quite those terms). Control of the finances on a day-to-day basis was essential; to that end it was necessary to appoint someone to keep a close eye on the accounts.

At each of the three institutions, the same man was chosen, and as the mid-point of the 19th century approached, Samuel Wing found himself clerk to the visiting justices, clerk to the governors of the infirmary and clerk to the guardians of the poor.

He attended the meetings of each of the committees, making recommendations on financial control and sometimes having to write letters to himself in the course of correspondence between the three bodies that he served.

Samuel Wing's duties at the asylum included a weekly visit in which he scrutinised the household books and drew up the accounts. It was the kind of task which he seems to have relished and within a short time of his appointment, he presented his masters with a list of some 20 books and ledgers which he considered essential for the proper financial management of the institution.

CHAPTER SEVEN

The Commissioners in Lunacy: 1845-53

Two Acts of Parliament were passed in 1845;* both were the work of Lord Ashley, later the Earl of Shaftesbury.

The legislation was the culmination of a battle which had been fought between Ashley and his followers and Edwin Chadwick, the secretary to the Poor Law Commissioners. Kathleen Jones† summarises the argument as follows:

> "The real point at issue between the Poor Law authorities and the Lunacy authorities was the old one of cure or detention. If the county asylums were looked upon as curative institutions, then their high cost was justified and they had a legitimate grievance against the Poor Law authorities for refusing to send them pauper lunatics who were susceptible to treatment. If . . . they were regarded merely as places of detention, the Poor Law authorities could rightly claim that they could do this work much more cheaply."

One important effect of the new legislation was to establish a permanent full-time Lunacy Commission, whose duty it was to inspect all asylums at least once every year and to deliver to the Lord Chancellor their annual reports as to the condition of the asylums and of the patients therein. Those appointed included five laymen (of whom Lord Ashley was one), plus three medical and three legal commissioners.

The medical commissioners were Thomas Turner, H. H. Southey, and J. R. Hume. The lawyers were James Mylne, John Hancock Hall and Bryan Procter ("better known as 'Barry Cornwall', the writer" – Jones). The commissioners visited in pairs; one doctor and one lawyer, and each of them recorded his

---

* 8 & 9 Vict. c.100 and c.126.

† Jones, K. A., *A history of the mental health services* – see Bibliography.

comments in the visitors' journal at the Bedford asylum at various times.

In their annual report to the Lord Chancellor in 1846 the commissioners included an account of their views on the "moral" treatment of the insane, which had not, it seems, been defined previously. They said that it consisted of:

> ". . . all those means which, by operating on the feelings and habits, exert a salutory influence, and tend to restore them to a sound and natural state."

They saw the abolition of virtually all forms of restraint – chains, manacles and leg irons etc. (as at the York Retreat) as an important part of their duty and their entries in the visitors' journal at the Bedford asylum bear witness to their determination to see that this was done. They had found that in the county asylums, whenever mechanical restraint had been discarded, there was a proportional improvement in the condition of the patients.

Those views were shared by many of the visiting magistrates at Bedford (although when the commissioners visited John Harris's private asylum as late as 1851 and recommended the removal of the chains and other fixtures on some of the beds there,* Harris was reluctant to do so without some way of controlling his more difficult patients).

James Reed, one of the visiting justices, noted in 1840:

> "One subject . . . having previously attempted to cut his throat, was confined to his bed but was making favourable progress – found one female very violent and frantic in her gestures and her language coarse and blasphemous."

Mr. Reed was accompanied on this visit by Edward Griffiths, who was evidently of less acute hearing and vision; *he* declared himself ". . . very much pleased and even gratified by everything I saw. Nothing could be more complete and perfect in every respect."

When the resident surgeon at the York Retreat, John Thursram, looked round the asylum, he found general cleanliness and order and made no comment on any measures of restraint but was critical of the overcrowding of the men – not only in the single yard, but in

---

* See Appendix IV, Nigel Lutt's account of the Springfield Asylum.

the beds in the galleries. Pither told him that it was because of the building operations then in progress, but the visitor regarded these conditions as very objectionable "both in a moral and physical point of view".

Thomas Charles Higgins found one man in handcuffs and nearly naked and was informed that the man wouldn't allow any clothes to remain on him if he were not so confined. Higgins suggested that ". . . some experiment might be made to entice him to better conduct", but (perhaps wisely), did not elaborate.

When the first official inspection of the Bedford asylum took place on January 9th 1845, Messrs. Southey and Hancock Hall found very few patients under physical restraint, and then only those who were very violent.

By 1845, three divisions had been formed, by way of classification, among the male patients:

1. "For those most noisy and troublesome."
2. "For those less so."
3. "For idiots" – i.e. the mentally handicapped.

A fourth division was added to the classification of the female patients; those considered fit to undertake needlework. There is no evidence, however, that this activity had been reintroduced by William Pither, whose dispute with Dr. Yeats in the matter of lace-making [p. 36] may have been long forgotten.

The commissioners suggested that the justices consider acquiring extra land "to afford more constant occupation for the male patients" and a further three acres were subsequently purchased.

When the commissioners visited the asylum on February 26th 1847 they found overcrowding at the institution; there were 191 inmates (93 men and 98 women). Nine patients were under restraint and 35 receiving medical treatment for physical illness. Since their visit the previous year, 71 patients had been admitted and 46 discharged; there had been 31 deaths.

A steady rise in the population of Bedford had taken place; the 1831 census had produced a total of about 7,000 and that of 1841, just over 9,000. Now, in 1847, there were about 10,000.

The Bedford Poor Law Union, the workhouse, whose infirmary ultimately became the North Wing of Bedford General Hospital, received paupers from 44 parishes with a total population of 31,759.

The Bedfordshire Directory for that year noted "a great influx of strangers with large families to gain the benefit of the free schools – open to all who become resident householders in Bedford".

A weekly corn and cattle market was held every Saturday on the north side of the Great Ouse* and the pig market took place on Mondays on the south side of the river.

The population, especially the women and children, were "much employed in the manufacture of straw and lace . . . a considerable trade in corn was transported *via* the Ouse to Lynn Regis, whence coal and other necessities were received in turn". One development in transport was to affect the affairs of the asylum; a branch line of the London and North Western railway was opened on November 18th 1846 after George Stephenson [of "Rocket" fame] and others had successfully argued the advantages of rail over water for the transport of goods at a meeting in the Mayor's parlour.

The railway line ran in close proximity to the back of the asylum grounds and became a popular escape route for some of those inmates who had become weary of their confinement. Much of the outer wall still remains intact, and separates the line from what is now a housing precinct and school playground. John Harris expressed concern, in his report of October 10th 1846, that ". . . the late heavy rains have retarded the erection of the wall between the asylum garden and the railway". One man, John Brown, was later recorded as having stripped himself naked and running a considerable distance along the railway line before the keepers were able to overtake him.

Sometimes the most ingenious escape techniques were adopted; a patient named Lenton slept in a cell, the door of which was fastened by a spring lock. The officer responsible for closing up one night found that the key wouldn't turn in the lock and assumed that the door was already fastened. It was found that Lenton had inserted a nail in the slot for the bolt of the door, which effectively prevented its closure.

The use of methods of physical restraint was not abandoned without a struggle and it may have been the case that John Harris,

---

* The cattle market was moved to Cople in 1989 amid protests from the farming community and was replaced by a housing development.

despite his worthy aspirations when he was first appointed, had some sympathy with the staff who had to cope with violent or suicidal patients as well as would-be escapees.

In 1847, one of the visiting justices, D. C. Cooper, "observed a man in manacles and fetters but was told he was apt to be mischievous". He suggested the provision of padded cells for violent patients as "padded bedsteads do not seem to be sufficient".

T. C. Higgins found Mary Ann Gibbs confined by her arms and legs; she was reputed to be very violent. "It would be well," he wrote, "if means could be devised that she could have her liberty without endangering her own life or the life of others." Later he "wondered how patients of such violent habits are restrained in other institutions without having the legs and arms confined". Nevertheless, in December 1848, Higgins noted that some destructive patients without the leather muffs were confined to their cells and expressed doubts: "It is a question whether their treatment be better than use of the muffs".

Marlborough Pryor, a JP for Herts and Middlesex, gave his opinion that the heavily barred windows gave "a great air of dullness and too much like a prison". Building works were in progress at the time but there were still no padded cells. He would also have liked to have seen more amusements for the patients and suggested "rocking horses in the yards and a few common books and papers within doors".

When John Harvey went round one evening at 6.30 he noted that some of the women patients had already gone to bed "having been placed in a warm bath", and the Kempston surgeon, Henry Littledale "regretted to observe one woman, under restraint and fastened to a bench – but she is described as destructive of . . . windows so as probably may justify this objectionable habit". Later, Harvey found two women fastened into padded beds because of their violent attempts at self-destruction.

The visiting justices and the commissioners were also concerned about the strong bars on the windows; suicide was fairly common and the most frequent method was employed by James Baker. The coroner's jury at the inquest into his death in January 1849 found that "the deceased strangled himself by hanging, being at the time insane". He had made a slipknot in his neckerchief and fastened it to one of the window bars.

The annual inspection by the commissioners in 1850 provoked much noise and turbulence particularly in the female refractory ward, where the overcrowding of the asylum was especially evident. (So much so that they recommended improving the air in the dayrooms by installing some ventilators opening into the chimneys.)

The total number of inmates had now risen to **252** and there had been 99 admissions in the previous year. There had been 40 deaths (from epilepsy, tuberculosis, old age and various other causes) and 17 patients were currently under medical treatment:

> "We learn on enquiry that seven patients are fastened to their beds by wrist locks at night and two appear to be frequently under the restraint of muffs. . . ."

The commissioners made no mention of "the Irishman, John Smith" who, it appears from the medical journal (which was begun in 1845, after the passage of the Lunacy Act of that year) was kept in leg and arm locks continually for some years. His name appeared in the journal until April 1852 after which he was mentioned no more.

The journal, in the statutory form, was produced for inspection by the commissioners at each of their visits. Apart from the data and the numbers of patients, male and female, other columns were provided for:

- The names of patients under restraint and under seclusion, by what means and for what period.
- The names of the patients under medical treatment.
- Report on the state of health of the patients and the condition of the asylum. (This column was usually left blank, or completed with some such comment as "good, in general" or "satisfactory".)
- Deaths, injuries and violence to patients.

This final column seems to have appealed most to the doctors, whose entries were sometimes almost enthusiastic:

February 7th 1848: "On 31st.ult. Ann Leckings struck one of the patient and one of the attendants and hurt them severely and she was put under restraint for a short time." (A strait-waistcoat for 12 hours.)

April 10th 1848: "Joseph West . . . attempted suicide by lacerating himself very much. He is [in] a precarious state very old and very weak." Seven days later his name had been moved to another column; he was in muffs and leg locks.

May 12th 1851 was an unfortunate time for some: "Henry East has given Henry Wright a black eye. Wm. Hardy has given Henry Smith a black eye." Then in July the aforesaid Henry East threw a stone at J. Norris and cut his face, finally turning his attention to William Smith and William Ganes in November. "He is unsafe to be at liberty," wrote Benjamin Matthews, the resident doctor, but East was not put under restraint – the commissioners had brought their powers to bear on such matters only a few months earlier:

On February 11th 1851, the commissioners, J. W. Mylne and S. Gaskell, set out in detail the rules for the future. There were 260 patients in the asylum, well clad, but some of the women were in strong dresses made of mattress ticking – that was to be stopped. The establishment was now lit by gas, which was a great improvement, and the commissioners were pleased to learn that a chapel and a new laundry were shortly to be added.

From the medical journal they had learned that eight patients were subject to restraint at various times but on enquiry they were told that several others were restrained for short periods "to prevent them from falling out of their chairs". They were not entirely convinced and ordered that every such instance be recorded with a view to diminishing the use of mechanical constraint:

- All rings and staples were to be removed from the walls of bedrooms and airing courts and from the seats in the dayrooms, as well as from the bedsteads. Restraining chairs to be converted into *leaning* chairs suitable for epileptics.
- Iron gates and strong bars to be removed "as far as possible".
- The instruments of restraint to be taken "in great measure, if not entirely out of the hands of the attendants" to some central point under the control of the resident medical officer or the matron.
- No nurses or attendants to be engaged unless they could read and write. Instruction in reading and writing was to be given forthwith to any already in post who needed it.
- A complete code of rules and regulations was to be drawn up for the instruction of the attendants in their conduct towards the patients.

- Some system of night-watching to be introduced and a record kept each night.
- A few leaning chairs to be installed for the aged, feeble, paralytic or sick. Better lavatories were to be provided.
- Constant efforts should be made to prevent the patients from *crouching* in the day rooms and airing courts and to provide encouraging occupations in keeping with their capacity.
- Each patient should be provided at dinner with a spoon or a knife and fork and *each* should have a vessel for whatever beverage was supplied with the meal.

> The commissioners added a parting shot: "We think that the female patients should be employed in making straw bonnets for their use and that they should be provided with shawls so that they may have the opportunity of taking exercise beyond the walls of the institution."

The commissioners were not alone in their concern to see that the patients were treated as humanely as consideration of their own and others' safety allowed. In 1848 Henry Littledale, the Kempston surgeon, commented:

> "A child of seven years of age sent from St. Albans appears scarcely a fit subject for the institution and the persons in charge observe nothing particularly indicative of want of intellect about her."

Mr. Higgins ordered an enquiry into the matter [but there is no record of the outcome].

The Rev. C. C. Beaty Pownall, vicar of Milton Ernest, was a prominent member of the committee of visiting justices and his entries in the visitors' journal bear eloquent witness to the extra *gravitas* which he brought to some of the more mundane problems at the asylum.

What Thomas Chalk called a "very close smell" in one of the men's galleries [sleeping quarters] where he found all the windows shut at three o'clock in the afternoon, Beaty Pownall referred to as "an unpleasant effluvium". On another occasion he wrote:

> "In a dark closet on the men's side called 'the bathroom' there is

an inconvenient and dangerous aperture in the floor which I think it would be very desirable to have covered over."

At a visit in 1851 he "... found the girl Burgess (who I am told is apt to be mischievous and troublesome) in the padded room – she was liberated on promising better behaviour", a course of action which the Rev. Henry Tatham must have applauded.

In January 1853, it was reported to the justices that William Smith, alias William Dubberly, had escaped from the asylum garden and:

"... proceeded across the fields in the direction of the river, two ward attendants being in close pursuit ... he then attempted to cross the river and being a good swimmer was enabled notwithstanding the rapid current nearly to reach the opposite shore when he suddenly disappeared and is supposed drowned."

An extensive search was made for the unfortunate man's body but without success; it was to be some weeks before it eventually surfaced. The justices decided that no blame was to be attached to the ward attendants.

CHAPTER EIGHT

An end in sight: 1852

By 1852, the asylum had been in existence for 40 years; it had been designed to hold 40 patients and now had to cope with 270. Despite the addition of extra sleeping galleries, dayrooms, yards and a bathhouse and laundry, the accommodation was quite inadequate and produced adverse comments from the commissioners and visiting justices – the poor ventilation led to dampness and foul air.

When John Harvey visited in the company of the new house steward, Mr. Upstone, and the matron, the idiot ward was particularly offensive: the steward asserted that it was "necessary to keep those patients very much warmer than the rest". Harvey was not particularly impressed and directed that holes be made in one of the doors to create a through draught. Similar problems in the female dayroom caused him to press for it to be rebuilt – the roof was, he said, too low. Another visitor, Charles Payne, suggested what he described as a much less expensive course of action, i.e. making "four or more apertures in the ceiling which might be closed at night before the patients went to bed on the floor above". That was just as good as a higher ceiling, he maintained.

Sleeping galleries for a further 70 patients were added, starting in 1848 and being followed by other smaller improvements but the building works produced some problems in themselves. T. C. Higgins complained that there were "workmen everywhere, in all parts of the asylum causing much dirt and confusion", and he was greatly alarmed at the encounter with one of the male patients, who was carrying "a large hammer in his hand, which had been carelessly left about by one of the workmen".

On August 2nd 1848, George Livius recorded the fact that ". . . a very serious complaint has been made respecting the conduct of one of the contractors, Thomas Bryant, towards some of the female patients".

The matter was investigated in the presence of John Harris, Mr.

Matthews, and Pither and his wife, the matron. There was no doubt that Bryant "had taken gross liberties with three of the female patients [who were named]". No further steps were taken on this occasion as the case was to be submitted to the magistrates on the following Tuesday. However, Harris felt it his duty to discharge Bryant from the premises and informed his son of the fact.

By January 1849 the new sleeping galleries had been in use for four months, and there were, in addition, two new dayrooms, two extra airing yards and two washhouses plus a new kitchen. The total number of patients was **236**, of whom 127 were female. In the autumn of that year John Harris suggested to one of the visitors, Boteler Smith, that certain additional works were required before the frosts set in. Mr. Smith authorised the supply of the lower galleries on each side with hot water by extending the existing piping and other minor improvements.

A month later Beaty Pownall noted with approval that that had been done but added his own suggestions, drawing attention to the fact that ablution facilities were deficient – on one floor there was only one such facility for 78 patients. During that same visit, he noticed a woman, Faith Sargeant, lying dead, "having expired the previous day".

Henry Littledale, the Kempston surgeon who was always on the alert for signs of lack of consideration for the patients, wrote that: "... I never visit the asylum without regret that the want of a walk or sufficient fences to surround the entire premises must deprive many of the inmates of some degree of liberty which might ... be returned to them." When he found Mary Ann Fleckney in a padded room and asked why, he was told that "she was kept there only when troublesome and not for any lengthy period".

While John Harvey was on his rounds, accompanied by Upstone, "Ann Impey was served with a violent paroxysm of fury and seized one of the patients by the throat. It required several of the assistants to convey her to the padded bed, where she was strapped down".

In February 1852, Upstone came to Harvey and Littledale (both of whom had expressed doubts about the amount of nature of the restraints still in use) and "tendered the resignation of himself and his wife, which we recommend the committee to accept". Benjamin Matthews, the resident house surgeon, and the assistant matron were appointed on a temporary basis to act in their place and in fact continued to do so for many months, earning general commendation for their efficiency.

Thomas Charles Higgins reported in March that ". . . the whole [is] indeed in as good a state as I have usually seen it", while Henry Littledale was delighted to find that there were no male patients under restraint. One woman was, however, confined in a cell, having been "spiteful and bitten one of the attendants". Samuel Hill, the superintendent of the asylum of the North Riding of Yorkshire, was very favourably impressed, and made particular note of the fact that all the duties had been conducted in the absence of the steward and of the matron.

Although much less physical restraint was now in use at the Bedford asylum, there was an admitted shortage of occupational and recreational facilities, particularly for the women.

Commissioners B. W. Procter and T. Turner at their annual visit of inspection in 1852 suggested that:

> ". . . a few cheap weekly publications not of a religious character should be added to the Bible, prayer books and tracts which at present constitute the stock of amusement provided for the patients." (Bryan Procter was, of course, the novelist Barry Cornwall.)

They were pleased to find at their next visit that "a supply of weekly periodical publications of a light and amusing kind has been procured for circulation among the patients".

The near abandonment of physical restraint was not without its price; Matthews blamed the "peculiar state of the weather" in February 1852 for the fact that some of the patients were more noisy and troublesome than usual. Higgins elicited from him the information that two women in particular had caused damage amounting to £15 since the new matron had been appointed the previous July: Gibbs was very mischievous – "I fear from what I learn that she will be the cause of injury to some patient or servant . . . Fowler seems to be very wasteful in destroying bed things and linen". Some plan must be devised to save the public property. Mr. Higgins was of the opinion that "the greatest evil to be contended against is the management of violent and mischievous patients . . . it is incredible what daily loss is sustained and it has become an intolerable burden".

On the occasion of a visit by Mr. Higgins in February 1853, Matthews was not able to accompany him on his round because he was in Bedford in consequence of the discovery of the body of W. T. Dubberly [see p. 99] who had been drowned 10 weeks before. Higgins directed that an accurate list of the patients be drawn up in order that he might visit *all 267* of them at his next visit. A pencilled note shows that he did so a week later but (no doubt from fatigue) he was otherwise silent.

In the winter of 1852, the visiting magistrates commissioned a survey and recommendations for improvements from Samuel Hill, the superintendent of the North and East Ridings of Yorkshire Asylum – it was considered, they said, "a perfect model of a curative lunatic asylum and Mr. Hill himself a most judicious exponent of all the requirements which an institution of the kind demands". Mr. Hill was accompanied by George Fowler Jones, a York architect, and they recorded their findings on December 6th.

Samuel Hill reported at considerable length:

> He began by expressing his general views on the control of difficult patients; especially consideration should be given to individual variations but he stressed the importance of "moral" treatment, as it had been promulgated at the York Retreat half a century before.* "Sympathy, sound discretion and firmness were required, and the patients had no longer to learn that punishment was the only reward for misconduct." His terms of reference, he said, didn't allow him to pursue "this interesting metaphysical subject" further (a constraint for which the more pragmatic recipients of his wisdom may have been grateful) but he had perhaps said enough "to explain his reasons for his recommendations *which by implication shew the unfitness of your asylum for the abode of its inmates*".
>
> Some patients were accommodated upstairs at night in dormitories but more were in single compartments, while others slept in single rooms on the ground floor. Some of the latter "communicated only with the open air into the airing

* He was preaching to the converted, as we have seen. Not only the commissioners, but successive medical officers and the visiting justices themselves, were well aware of the principles involved, although ensuring that they were practised was another matter.

yards"; he hoped that these weren't used at night but suspected that "the temptation to do so was not always overcome".

The two wings (north-west and south-east) were at so low a level as to render efficient ventilation impracticable – cold air was admitted through gratings in the walls, and in some rooms there were no fireplaces. The hot water warming apparatus was quite useless.

The ventilation system also came in for criticism: ". . . the perpendicular shafts for the escape of foul air act in the opposite manner and admit cold blasts into the sleeping rooms. . . ." Some areas were warmed by Perkins's hot water apparatus but on the occasion of Samuel Hill's visits certain of the furnaces were under water, "the springs being unusually full".

The flagstones in the day-rooms were "a most objectionable flooring for women without shoes and stockings to stand upon . . .". The windows were too high so that the patients couldn't see out without climbing on to the tables or forms. In the original central block [designed by John Wing in 1811] the rooms were better than those in the later wing but their use had been appropriated to purposes other than those intended – one was now a pump-and-scullery room, for example.

The chapel was on the men's side of the building and was approached by a staircase far too small for "the numbers of patients who ought to attend Divine Service when the asylum is increased in size". Two infirmary wards were needed for the sick, the aged and the infirm.

Dr. Hill now turned to his proposed improvements and alterations, and was unable to resist a small homily by way of preface: "In order to govern with mercy you must construct with judgement – you must not have the dark corners, obscure recesses closed with doors, blockaded windows. . . ." If the disordered senses were pent up, they would not quit if this were continued. The patients should be able to look beyond the high dead walls through light and agreeable palisading which would afford all the safety necessary by having it seven feet high and on "a dwarf wall".

He had special reasons for the site he had chosen for the residence of the superintendent; he was persuaded that "all future arrangements should be so made as to cause the

> superintendent to pass much more frequently through the various parts of the establishment in which the patients are distributed". [No ivory tower for him!]
>
> The detailed estimates of the costs of the improvements suggested by Samuel Hill included those for a house for the superintendent (£2,010), single-bedded rooms, corridors, bathrooms, four day rooms 40 x 18 feet with associated dormitories and lavatories (£2,850), all in a south-east extension. He also proposed two new wings, a lodge, a new archway and gates and iron palisading for the walls. His estimate for all this amounted to £17,000.

The architect, George Fowler Jones, who presented detailed plans for the extensions, added a much shorter report on the general state of repair of the existing buildings:

> Extensive re-roofing was required: "... the roofs over the chapel and south-east wings or those recently built have been I fear erected with greater regard to small cost than durability . . . I may state that I found the ventilation everywhere defective, the paved floors of the lower day rooms and cells damp and ... the walls everywhere streaming with wet."

The response of the committee of visiting magistrates to these reports was an immediate acceptance, with the estimates, subject to the approval of the Secretary of State. Their colleagues in Herts. and Hunts. were to be asked to add their authorisation and to agree to raise the necessary funds "by mortgage or otherwise" in the following proportions:

- Bedfordshire; two-fifths (£6,800).
- Hertfordshire; two-fifths (£6,800).
- Huntingdonshire; one-fifth (£3,400).

At their annual visit on December 21st 1952, the commissioners, Messrs. B. W. Procter and T. Turner noted simply that they understood "that a large sum is about to be laid out in enlarging and improving the institution". Their opinion, and that of the Secretary of State, was not recorded, but the visiting justices evidently felt the need to defend the continued local situation (and control) of the asylum. At their monthly meeting on January 3rd 1853 they urged:

> "... the extreme importance of the grant now demanded. The

> cost ought not to weigh as a feather in the scale against the sacred obligation of administering to the necessities of those individuals who are affected with the sorest malady incident to human nature; and who can forbear evincing his own gratitude for the exemption of such an evil by cheerfully contributing his mite towards the mitigation of the calamity in others?"

The visitors were "not without hope" that the scheme would also be to the advantage of the rate-payers themselves; the increased accommodation would ensure a greater number of patients with a reduction in the consequent weekly cost per head. And so, it was asserted, the institution would gradually become self-supporting!

Among other unstated advantages to the rate-payers of the three counties, who shared the expenses of the Bedford asylum, would be that with the reduction in the weekly cost of maintenance there would be "less temptation to evade the law by detaining idiots (the mentally handicapped), however harmless, from partaking of the advantages offered to them at the asylum on moderate terms".

It had been calculated that the addition of a farthing, "or nearly so", to the rates would be sufficient for the first year's instalment and interest.

These arguments, and any discussions that went unrecorded, failed to convince their colleagues, and two weeks later, the Court of Quarter Sessions appointed a special committee, with Thomas Charles Higgins in the chair, to draw up proposals "in respect of the arrangement most desirable for the purchase of land and the erection of a new asylum thereon . . .".

The committee included Marlborough Pryor, representing Hertfordshire, and William Williams, the mayor of Bedford, who spoke for the Borough.

Their first meeting had to be postponed because a new application had been submitted; Cambridgeshire now wanted to join with the original three in building an asylum for all four counties, the cost being shared among them. The initial approach had been made in the form of a letter from the clerk of the committee of visitors of Cambridgeshire, the Isle of Ely and the Borough of Cambridge, who had combined in a union to establish and manage a pauper lunatic asylum for all three.

A delegation from Cambridge put their case at the meeting in

February 1853 and as a result, it was agreed by all the parties to recommend that a new asylum be built. Two hundred acres of land should be purchased "as near as may be to the Great Northern Railway* at a cost of £70,000 and that the counties of Hertford, Cambridge and Huntingdon should be invited to unite with Bedford county for the purpose".

The proposals were agreed at the next quarter sessions, although the mayor opposed them on behalf of the Borough Council who "viewed with alarm" the intention to spend such a sum to build a new asylum. Mr. E. Eagles† had written to the mayor in the name of the county rate-payers, who were no doubt alarmed at the prospect of losing valuable county assets if a new asylum were built elsewhere.

Commissioners J. W. Milne and J. R. Hume made an extra visit a month later and while they noted without comment that there was "a prospect for further accommodation from all the three united counties", added:

> "We learn, however, that the scheme at one time entertained of these counties being combined with Cambridgeshire in the erection of a new asylum is not likely to be adopted – a result which for many reasons we think is not to be regretted."

Negotiations dragged on through the summer of 1853. In May, David King, the clerk to the Cambridge visitors, wrote to say that they wanted to hear "something conclusive" with regard to the intentions of the other three. The matter should be settled at once or "... I fear the chance of our County, Isle and Borough uniting [with the others] will be at an end". He had earlier indicated that they wouldn't be able to take any steps towards implementing the proposals without consultations with a view to dissolution of their existing union.

Theed Pearse, the town clerk, wrote in August to record the continued opposition of his Council:

> ". . . we cannot but express our astonishment that such a

---

* James Collett-White suggests that this railway line suited all except the Cambridge delegates, being convenient to all three for the safe transport of their patients in groups.

† Ezra Eagles was the coroner for the Borough of Bedford.

> resolution should under [the] circumstances have been proposed, seconded and carried, a Bill having been introduced into the House of Commons . . . giving the ratepayers control over the expenditure of the county stock. . . ."

Inevitably, the question of compensation to the county for the loss of its assets was raised. Bedford proposed the appointment of an independent arbitrator; Cambridge refused categorically – they had, they said, no legal powers to make such payments.

At the adjourned quarter sessions on August 29th, it was proposed by John Harvey and seconded by Lord Charles James Fox Russell* that the existing union of the three counties be extended to include the county of Cambridge:

> ". . . it being distinctly understood that the question of compensation in regard of any loss to be sustained by the present Union [of the three counties] be referred to arbitration."

That brought all further discussion to an end; a motion put to the committee of visitors of the Cambridgeshire, Isle of Ely and Borough of Cambridge lunatic asylum, that their union be dissolved, was lost by six votes for and seven against. There would be no Four Counties Asylum and the way was now clear for preparations for the other three to go ahead with plans for a new institution with room for 600 patients on 200 acres of ground as close as possible to the Great Northern Railway. The Three Counties asylum was ultimately built at Arlesey, which met this requirement.

* The Russell family were great supporters of the radical Whigs, as were the Whitbreads.

CHAPTER NINE

The final stages: 1853-56

In 1853, the Bedford asylum held on average about **270** patients, with a slight preponderance of women. [By 1857 this figure had reached 323.] Those in the household numbered 34, including the resident medical officer, Benjamin Matthews (salary £100 plus a gratuity of £45), the matron, Mrs. Anna Galer (£36.5s.0d.) and a storekeeper/chief ward attendant – the steward – (£33.16s.0d.). The total income of the institution for the year amounted to £6,176.19s.4d. and the total of outgoing payments to £6,222.17s.9d.

These, and many other details were contained in the printed annual financial statement.* By 1853, the three counties plus the Borough of Bedford had combined in a union which managed the existing asylum, sharing the income and costs *pro rata*.

Beer was brewed on the premises – 14,366 gallons over the course of the year – at 6¾d. per gallon, which included payment to the un-named brewer who was employed in the task for 68 days (at 3s. a day). Vinegar and other condiments cost £8.19s.0d. but the visitors were able to save money by purchasing British wine at only £1 per dozen bottles; their three dozen came to a mere £3. Among the miscellaneous items were "cricket and foot balls", while music for different kind of patients' ball cost fifteen shillings.

Rates and taxes came to £41.0s.2d. which included two "improvement rates". The drug bill was for £17.5s.0d. which was somewhat less than that for wine – British or not – and spirits (£24.3s.3d.).

Most of the men were employed in the garden or on the farm, but as Henry Littledale observed, the women were without work of any kind. His comment was noted and shortly afterwards the commissioners were told that 51 female patients were occupied in

* The statement for the year 1853 is reproduced in facsimile as Appendix IV.

household tasks in the workroom or in the laundry. His satisfaction was somewhat tempered, however, by his finding some men working in the laundry. Dr. Denne, the new resident medical superintendent, who was appointed in 1854, explained that it was the height of the boilers that had caused him to employ men for that purpose!

Another visitor, Mr. William St. Quentin, was similarly outraged to find two male patients at work there – "one turning the mangle and the other taking clothes out of the copper". Denne was able to reassure him, however; he was "gradually breaking in some of the females to turn the mangle". Furthermore, he had a plan regarding the boilers "by which the assistance of male patients may be entirely dispensed with". That appears to have reassured the justices.

The arrival of William Denne and of his wife, who took over as matron, signalled the final elimination of all forms of physical restraint from the Bedford asylum. Mr. Higgins wrote a testimonial for the out-going matron:

> "On behalf of the Visitors of the Bedford Lunatic Asylum I desire to recommend Mrs. Anna Galer for the office of matron of the Buckinghamshire Asylum. Mrs. Galer is highly respectable and has had now considerable experience in the management of the asylum. She leaves in consequence of the appointment of a resident medical officer whose wife is necessarily the matron."

John Harris had continued as superintendent but was non-resident, and had moved to Springfield House when he opened his private asylum in 1837. He attended the Bedford asylum every day and his assistant was resident there, but that arrangement was no longer acceptable. The negotiations over the new asylum had brought from the Commissioners in London several comments including the following:

> ". . . having regard to the most important questions of medical treatment and cure, the Commissioners in Lunacy much prefer asylums of moderate size i.e. 200 and not exceeding 300 patients under the charge of one medical officer and an assistant [both presumably resident]".

After discussions had taken place with John Harris it was decided to advertise two posts: resident medical superintendent and an assistant medical officer, who was also to live at the asylum. Harris himself was to retain the title of visiting surgeon. The justices had written to Lord Palmerston in May 1853 requesting an amendment to clause 57 of a bill which had been introduced into the House of Lords.* They wanted it to "empower a superannuation to be granted to Mr. Harris for his long service should he cease to be superintendent by law, or by any new arrangement. The letter pointed out that Harris's post as superintendent and visiting surgeon had been approved under the terms of the 1845 Act of Parliament [Vic. 8 & 9 c.126].

It is not clear whether the request was granted but William Denne became the new medical superintendent in 1854. His assistant, William Edward Musson, was also appointed. Denne wrote to Samuel Wing, the visiting justices' clerk, on September 27th.:

> "My dear Sir
>
> I yesterday forwarded a book of patterns of paper to you having selected those the numbers of which are on the enclosed sheet. . . . Mrs. Denne will go down to Bedford with me early in the next week and [as] there is so much to see about we propose staying the night . . .
>
> PS I have omitted Mr. Musson's bedroom (below) which I think will require papering, if so will you let him choose one. – W.D."

The particulars of William Denne's training and experience before his appointment are not available, but Musson's detailed application has survived† and provides an interesting glimpse of the training of a young doctor of the time. His hand-written covering letter reads:

> "To the Committee of Visitors Bedford Lunatic Asylum
>
> My Lords and Gentlemen
>
> I beg most respectfully to offer myself as a Candidate for the

---

* This was possibly the bill which resulted in the Lunatics Act of 1853 – Vict. 16 and 17 c.70 amended in c.96.

† County Record Office: ref. LB7/12.

vacant Appointment of Resident Medical Officer to the Bedford Lunatic Asylum –

I commenced the study of my profession at the age of 16 & have pursued it uninterruptedly to the present time. I am now in my 24th year – During the first two years I matriculated at the University of London, and acquired a knowledge of dispensing & general practice as an apprentice of Mr. Harris of 43 Gower St, Bedford Square, London. During my apprenticeship and afterwards as a student at St. Thomas's Hospital (where I was resident dresser and clinical clerk*) I had the management of numbers of cases of delirium tremens proceeding [from] both accidents in debilitated persons and from the influence of stimulating drinks & since I obtained my Diploma of College of Surgeons and Apothecaries' Hall I have been residing as assistant for two years with Mr. F. I. Bellingham, surgeon of Bourne having generally a great share, and sometimes the entire care, of a large district of Union, with a workhouse, where I have had the management of a number of cases of Lunacy, temporary and confirmed, prior to their removal to an asylum –

These particulars with the testimonials and certificates which I have the honor of laying before you, will, I trust, secure for me your kind consideration,

I have the honor to remain,
My Lords & Gentlemen
Your most obedient Servant
Wm.Edwd. Musson"

This letter was accompanied by three closely printed sheets of copies of testimonials and certificates, from the Treasurer to St. Thomas's Hospital (R. Bagallay), four of the surgeons and two of the physicians there,† plus a recommendation from R. G. Whitfield, Resident Medical Officer and Secretary to the hospital.

There were also testimonials from the surgeon Richard Harris, with whom Musson had served as apprentice before going on to St.

---

* A "dresser" worked in a team led by a surgeon, and a "clerk" in one whose chief was a physician.

† The surgeons were: Gilbert Mackmurdo F.R.S., Samuel Solly F.R.S., John Simon F.R.S. and F. Le Gros Clark (who was also a lecturer in surgical anatomy). The physicians were T. A. Barker M.D. and Jas. R. Bennett M.D.

Thomas's, and from F. J. Bellingham, for whom the applicant had been an assistant in his general practice for two years:

> "... I have great pleasure in bearing testimony to his general and professional ability, as well as to the moral rectitude of his character.... During his residence with me, he has several times been left in sole charge of the practice, and has always discharged the duties which then devolved upon him to my satisfaction. . . ."

Most of the documents referred specifically to the application to Bedford Lunatic Asylum, although some mentioned the post as that of "house surgeon". All commended him for his gentlemanly and humane character, his intelligence and industry and/or his general professional skill. He was, they said, "well-qualified", or even "exceedingly well qualified", to undertake the duties of the resident medical officer of the Bedford asylum and its 300 inmates. This is no reflection on them, or on him, but it underlines, perhaps, a widely held view of the nature of such institutions at the time. The medical expertise which Musson was expected to bring to the patients was that appropriate to general practice; he would prescribe for their bodily ailments and pronounce them dead, if they were so, but little more.

Some selected correspondence; 1854/5:

November 18 1854; From John Harvey; Ickwell Bury, to Samuel Wing:

> "My dear Sir,
>
> I have read a letter from Mr. Musson in which he expresses considerable dissatisfaction at the regulations relating to the duties of the assistant medical officer being *printed* as he fears it would degrade him in the opinion of the other members of the profession. Entre nous I was rather surprised at Mr. Musson having had the good sense to accept the office he holds after the very strong opinions which the other candidates for the appointment expressed on the subject and I am inclined to think he has reason on his side. He expresses no unwillingness but on the contrary anxiety to perform the duties but objects to a *printed* announcement of his doing so. . . ."

A telegram from John Harvey to the chairman of the asylum (T. C. Higgins) from Euston Station on August 8th 1854:

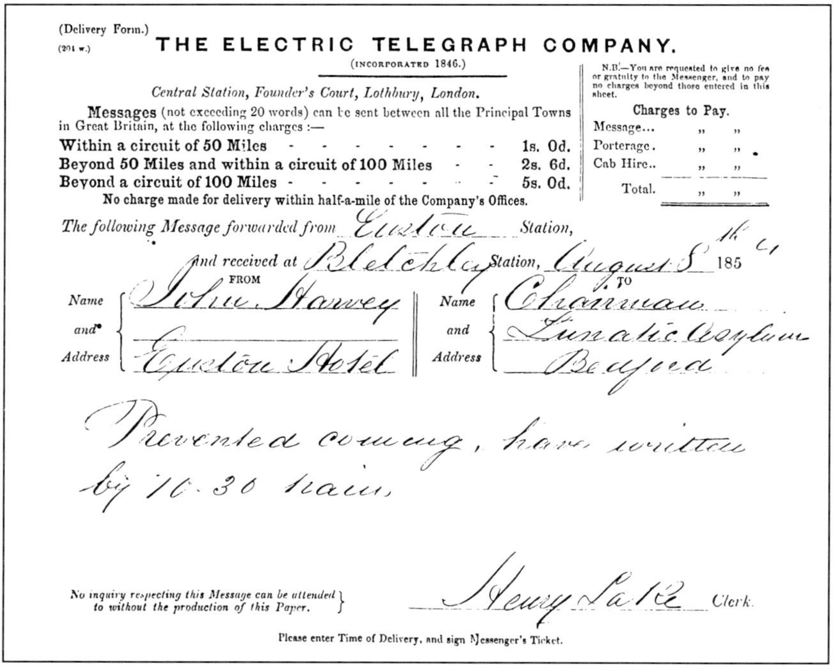
(Delivery Form.)
(201 w.)

THE ELECTRIC TELEGRAPH COMPANY.
(INCORPORATED 1846.)

Central Station, Founder's Court, Lothbury, London.

Messages (not exceeding 20 words) can be sent between all the Principal Towns in Great Britain, at the following charges :—

Within a circuit of 50 Miles	**1s. 0d.**
Beyond 50 Miles and within a circuit of 100 Miles	**2s. 6d.**
Beyond a circuit of 100 Miles	**5s. 0d.**

No charge made for delivery within half-a-mile of the Company's Offices.

N.B.—You are requested to give no fee or gratuity to the Messenger, and to pay no charges beyond those entered in this sheet.

Charges to Pay.

Message...	"	"
Porterage.	"	"
Cab Hire..	"	"
Total.	"	"

The following Message forwarded from Euston *Station,*

And received at Bletchley *Station,* August 8th 1854

FROM
Name and Address John Harvey, Euston Hotel

TO
Name and Address Chairman, Lunatic Asylum, Bedford

Prevented coming, have written by 10.30 train.

No inquiry respecting this Message can be attended to without the production of this Paper.

Henry Sale *Clerk.*

Please enter Time of Delivery, and sign Messenger's Ticket.

Telegram from John Harvey

The privately owned telegraph company was incorporated in 1846. It was not until the Telegraph Act of 1868 became law that the Postmaster General was allowed to take over (by purchase).

From Thos. Erskine Austin, clerk to the Luton Union (Beds. and Herts.) to Samuel Wing:

> "Dear Sir In reply to your letter . . . I beg to inform you that we have no Hertfordshire lunatic at present to send to the Bedford asylum but I shall be glad to hear of the first vacancy you have for a female who happens to belong to the wrong side of the street of the village of Markyate in the hamlet of Humbershoe [?] in the parish of Studham, Bedfordshire. . . ."

From William Denne to Samuel Wing: (8 Dec. 1854).

"Dear Mr. Wing,

It has just occurred to me I should have given notice of an escape which occurred here yesterday morning about 1/29 o'clock am. It was a female patient named Jane Tingwood she was retaken & brought back by two men who picked her up at the style [*sic*] crossing the fields towards Elstow – Do I read the Act right that notice ought to be given to the Commissioners cap 97 c.93?

Yours truly

Wm Denne"

(Denne had been in post for only six weeks and was still very conscious of the weight of the law governing his activities.)

From the clerk to the visiting justices of the prison [un-named] to Mr. W. S. Lutwidge, secretary to the Commissioners in Lunacy, at 19 Whitehall Place, London. The commissioners wanted assurance that a patient named Lucy Sharman had been "properly dealt with":

"April 4th 1855 Sir, I have the Honor to acknowledge the receipt of your letter of the 3rd. instant and will communicate to Mr. Denne yr. request in respect of Lucy Sharman. As Clerk to the Visiting Justices of the Prison I am acquainted more fully with the circumstances connected with this Patient. Lucy Sharman has been committed to Prison no less than 15 times for acts of insubordination or malicious injury to the workhouse of the St. Neots union situate at Eaton Socon in this county. The last offence, however, for which she was committed occurred at Bedford where she broke the window of the Relieving Officer & was sentenced to 21 days imprisonment. During her imprisonment however, upon this occasion she broke the window of her cell and was altogether so violent that the attention of the Surgeon was called to her case and after carefully watching it he came to the conclusion that Sharman was of unsound mind . . . the Relieving Officer made the usual application for her admission into the County Asylum.

Since her acception into the asylum Mr. Denne tells me she has been very industrious and well conducted . . . he will no doubt recommend her discharge as soon as he has satisfied himself of the Patient's sanity". [Copy – no signature]

From Marlborough Pryor (a Hertfordshire magistrate on the Bedfordshire union committee of visiting justices) to Samuel Wing, writing from Cromer, October 23rd 1854:

> He hoped to be at Weston the following week, "... after then I shall be ready to look over the proof sheets of the new General Rules and also the regulations and orders. . . ."

Samuel Wing to Mr. W. S. Lutwidge, secretary to the Commissioners:

> "November 6th 1854 – Immediate
> Sir, will you allow me to enquire whether Lord Palmerston has certified his approval of the New General Rules for the government of this asylum, and if so, that you will kindly procure their transmission to me by return of post* as we are about to commence the new system of management on Wednesday next and we may be placed in difficulty without them."

After much discussion and careful drafting by representatives of all three counties, the new general rules and regulations were agreed. An estimate for printing them was obtained from Mr. Grey of St. Mary's, in October 1854:

> "200 copies printed on good paper done up in printed wrappers
> – £8.0.0.
> 200 copies printed on good paper done up in cloth, gilt lettered on side
> – £13.0.0.
> 200 copies printed on good paper done up in leather and also gilt lettered
> – £14.0.0."

Among the duties laid down for the justices on the visitors' committee at their monthly meetings were those of examining the weekly returns, inspecting the food, and also "to see all the patients and all the wards . . . to examine and sign the medical and other

---

* November 6th 1854 was a Monday! A more notable example of the Home Department's confidence in the reliability of the postal service of the time is quoted by Stockdale in his account of Bedford Prison (p. 195 – see Bibliography). In March 1854 a man named Abel Burrows had been condemned to death; a respite arrived by post, the execution having been arranged for the following morning.

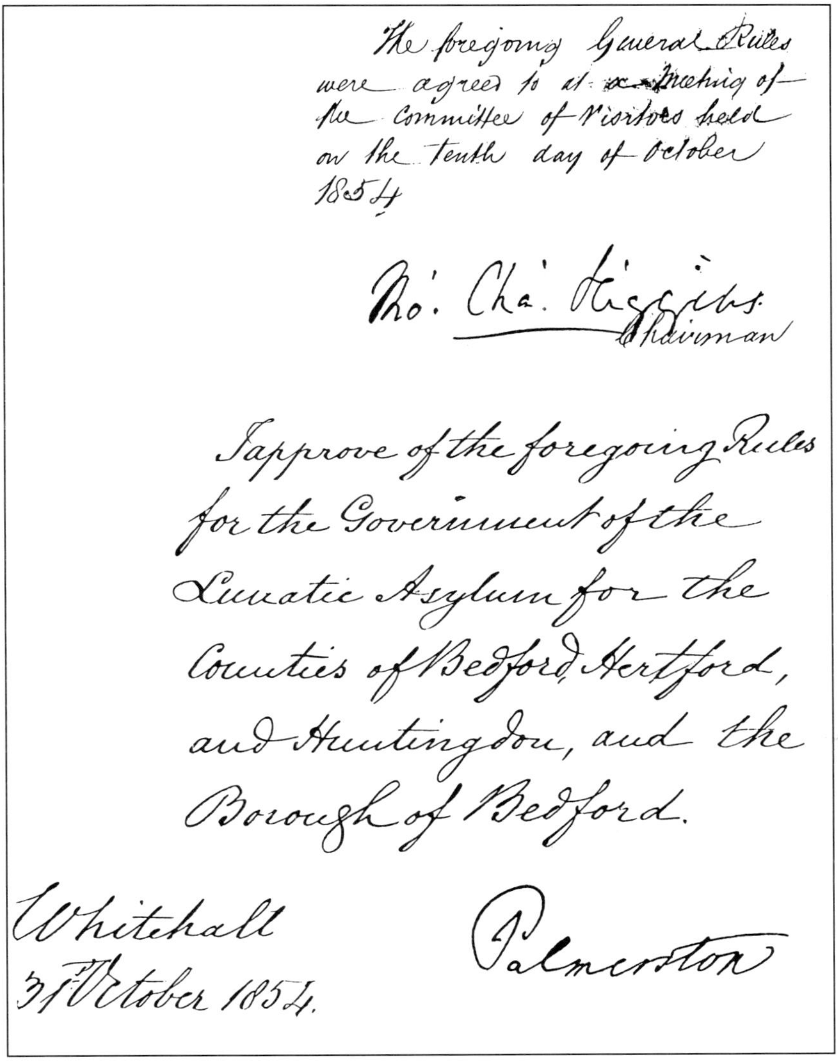
The foregoing General Rules were agreed to at a Meeting of the Committee of Visitors held on the tenth day of October 1854

Tho: Cha: Higgins. Chairman

I approve of the foregoing Rules for the Government of the Lunatic Asylum for the Counties of Bedford, Hertford, and Huntingdon, and the Borough of Bedford.

Whitehall 31st October 1854.

Palmerston

Palmerston's approval of the new regulations

journals" and to see every patient admitted since the previous meeting (unless the medical officer thought it might be harmful to him or her). No officer of the asylum except the visiting surgeon [John Harris], the chaplain and the clerk to the visitors [Samuel Wing] was allowed to have "any occupation unconnected with the asylum".

The annual audit of the accounts was to take place at the annual general meeting, when the report by the visiting justices on the state of the asylum to be presented to the next general quarter sessions was to be agreed.

Detailed regulations concerning the patients were specified in the document, eg:

> "XVIII. That the male and female patients be kept in separate wards and that no male attendant, servant or patient be allowed to enter the female wards or any female to enter the male wards, except in cases where the resident medical superintendant shall deem it advisable to appoint nurses or female servants for that purpose."
>
> "XIX. That no patient be struck or kept in perpetual restraint or seclusion . . . at any time except by medical authority . . . and further, that no forcible means shall be used for giving food or medicine but in the presence of the resident medical superintendant who shall at the time, record the fact in his journal."

Friends and relations were allowed to visit them once a fortnight, or more often in case of illness, in which case they might, if they couldn't attend on a weekday, visit exceptionally on a Sunday.

No dormitory for male patients was to contain fewer than three beds, and all male patients were to sleep in single beds.*

The escape of patients from the asylum was treated with as much seriousness as that of the inmates of the prison (whose regulations seem, indeed, to have provided the model for much of this section of the document), and discharges were closely controlled:

> "XXXII. That patients may be discharged in either of the following modes:
>
> 1. By an order of three of the visitors signified in writing under their hands and seals.
> 2. By warrant of Her Majesty, or of one of Her Majesty's principal Secretaries of State in the case of criminal lunatics."

Among the miscellaneous provisions was that of dismissal of any officer, ward attendant or servant receiving a fee or perquisite, either

* The regulations were silent on the question of the female patients' sleeping arrangements.

in money or in kind, from a tradesman, a patient or a patient's friend. The resident medical superintendent and all officers and servants were instructed "as far as possible and consistent with the performance of their respective duties, punctually to attend divine service in the chapel . . .".

The existence of a visiting surgeon was optional and, designed, of course to accommodate John Harris's appointment;* he was to "give such attendance . . . and perform other duties" as required by the regulations in force at the time.

The rules were much more specific with regard to the duties of the resident medical superintendent, and the regulations even more so:

1. He had to be a member of the Royal College of Surgeons, a Doctor of Medicine *or* a Fellow or Licentiate of the College of Physicians of London, Edinborough or Dublin and a Licentiate of the company of Apothecaries.
2. He was whole-time at the asylum and having no connection outside.
3. "He shall constantly reside in the asylum and shall never absent himself one night or more without the written consent of one of the Committee of Visitors. . . ."

The superintendent was responsible for general supervision and for the condition of the patients; he was accountable to the Committee for the management and condition of the establishment, and had the direction of "the medical, surgical and moral treatment of the patients". He superintended the performances† of the duties of the matron, steward, attendants and servants.

The chaplain was to be a clergyman of the established Church, in priest's orders and licensed by the Bishop of the diocese.

The matron should "obey the resident medical officer [as Mrs. Denne had in any case undertaken to do, without such qualification] in all matters relating to medical care, and treatment of the female patients".

---

* This may have been an indication that Lord Palmerston had not thought fit to amend the parliamentary bill in accordance with the request made earlier (p. 111).

† Evidently not as modern an expression as I had thought! – BC.

The rules ended with a section on general management:

> "XLVII. That as the cure, comfort, protection and security of the patients are the essential objects of the asylum; all the arrangements and regulations shall be made for their promotion and that therefore harshness in demeanour or language, violence in conduct, severity towards the patients, or neglect of the directions framed for their welfare and advantage, must ever be avoided by all the officers, attendants and servants employed in the establishment on pain of censure or dismissal; and that restraint and vehemence be superseded by that kind and constant vigilance on the part of the attendants, which shall protect the patient from danger and accidents, and shall prevent any escape, and that the attention of every officer, attendant and servant . . . shall be required to the provisions in the 71 and 77 sections of the act, 8 & 9 Vict. cap.126, as to the penalties on the escape of patients and punishment for their ill treatment, and which provisions the Committee of Visitors will duly enforce."

William Denne settled rapidly into his post and attracted favourable comments from visitors and commissioners alike. Henry Littledale was impressed by the suggestions for improvements that the superintendent put to him; he expressed the hope that some of them would be put into effect (without, of course, serious expenditure). No doubt the air of "cheerfulness and satisfaction" that he noticed among the patients had been helped by repairs to the rocking-horses, which he had earlier reported as being unfit for use: "I strongly recommend their restoration," he had written, "as very useful in the female department."

The commissioners, J. W. Mylne and S. Clarke, were pleased to find a perceptible improvement in the female patients at their annual inspection on July 13th 1855; the women were "more quiet, orderly and better dressed and occupied". But they recommended yet again the abandonment of the use of dresses made out of mattress ticking and that the women be supplied with bonnets, cloaks and shawls to allow them to get more outdoor exercise "especially beyond the limits of the premises".

Of the visiting justices, Thomas Charles Higgins was of the opinion that the women patients were more manageable than the men: ". . . I think a more numerous and better class of female servants are required – and the female patients require a more cheerful prospect around them – which can only be effected by removal of the high walls." He didn't seem to think that improvement appropriate for the men – probably because they were more likely to escape.

The commissioners agreed that the eight walled yards presented "a dull and cheerless and prison-like appearance". They were glad to find that the magistrates of Bedfordshire had decided to build a new county asylum subject to the concurrence of the third county, Huntingdonshire.

They did not consider expenditure on the existing fabric to be justified but "a liberal outlay might prudently and usefully be made in the articles of furniture, means of occupation, cheerful books and objects calculated to attract the attention or afford recreation and amusement to the patients".

They noted with approval that 11 chronic cases had been sent home on trial and had subsequently been discharged. Dr. Denne intended to relieve the establishment by removing several of the inmates "provided they can be judiciously taken care of at home or elsewhere".

Until the new asylum was built, pauper patients who couldn't be accommodated at Bedford might be sent to other public asylums e.g. to Bucks., Warwickshire or the Borough of Birmingham, who had some vacancies. If that wasn't possible, they suggested renting a suitable building near the asylum.

All the walls were to be lowered and some dividing walls were to be removed. The yards were to be planted and made either useful or ornamental. The commissioners ordered the removal of all bars and "wire-work" from the windows.

The justices were conscientious in their inspection of the food provided for the patients. John Harvey saw the dinner being prepared and tasted the plum pudding, which he pronounced excellent – as was the beer. Lynn Smart found the pudding to be good and wholesome, but suggested that it could be improved by the addition of "a few pounds of treacle in lieu of a portion of the raisins". He didn't agree with his colleague about the beer, though. It wasn't as good as it ought to have been, considering the quantity of malt and hops said to have been used in the brewing. A month later it was the turn of the Rev. C. C. Beaty Pownall to give an authoritative judgment on the quality of the beer. His visit took place in August and: "any fault to be found with it may be referred to the late close and highly electrical state of the weather". And that was the end of the matter.

In July 1855, Richard Gaunt, the oldest of the inmates, died. He had been admitted in 1814, two years after the asylum had been opened and he had then been said to be 65 years old. If that was correct, which is doubtful, he had survived until the age of 107! His death was soon to be followed by that of the institution in which he had spent the last 40 years of his life:

> "At a Meeting of the Committees severally appointed by the Counties of Bedford, Hertford and Huntingdon to provide an asylum for the said Counties and to proceed for that purpose in a manner by 'the Lunatic Asylums Act 1853' provided in the case of a County not having an asylum duly convened, and held at the Railway Hotel near to the Railway Station of the Great Northern Railway in the County of Hertford on Thursday the Twenty fifth day of October 1855.
>
> Present
>
> *For the County of Bedford*
> Thomas Charles Higgins Esquire
> William Lynn Smart Esquire
> Robert Lindsell Esquire
>
> *For the County of Hertford*
> William Franks Esquire
> Marlborough Pryor Esquire
>
> *For the County of Huntingdon*
> James Rust Esquire M.P."

Marlborough Pryor was elected chairman of the joint committee* and (perhaps by way of achieving a balance) the ubiquitous Samuel Wing was appointed as their clerk.

---

* C. Northcote Parkinson has pointed out that the term "committee" was originally singular, i.e. a person appointed to manage the affairs of a lunatic.

Preparations to build the new asylum for the three counties now began in earnest, but in the meantime the Bedford justices and the staff of their overcrowded institution had to cope as best they could. While Beaty Pownall was calling the roll in No. 4 ward:

> "... one patient (Samuel Newman) became very violent, struck another patient several times and was obliged to be removed to a separate apartment, which was effected with considerable difficulty ... the poor fellow having to be carried by main force struggling with 4 or 4 ward attendants [*sic* – Pownall was evidently under some strain at this point] the whole length of the House."

Patients continued to escape – John Norris was brought back on the following day but Jacob Reid remained at liberty for only three hours, and others succeeded in committing suicide. In June 1855, a coroner's jury found that Elizabeth Biggs "strangled herself by hanging, being at the time insane". Lynn Smart and his colleagues investigated the circumstances and concluded that there had been remissness on the part of Jane Prentice, the attendant who had special charge of the patient, and recommended that she be given leave of absence and then dismissed.

The Rev. Beaty Pownall wrote that:

> "a very distressing occurrence took place on Wednesday last in the asylum – the suicide of the storeman John Howes who has been in the institution not quite a fortnight. The jury's verdict was that the unfortunate man was of unsound mind at the time that he committed the act".

Mr. St. Quentin was told by Denne of the misconduct by three of the attendants in having put a patient (Charles Smith) into the bath with all his clothes on. Denne attributed this "act of wanton cruelty" to one of the three, Thomas Holmes, who was discharged on the spot after having been subjected to "a lecture". As he was to leave the same day, St. Quentin didn't think it necessary to press the matter further – presumably Holmes could have been prosecuted for assault. The other two received cautions only.

On May 31st 1856 Lynn Smart was happy to record that as the Crimean War had ended: "On the 29th inst. the males had a supper with a little beer and a pipe and the females had tea and plum cake and had the band of music to which they danced – they were all quite sensible that the treat was given to them to celebrate 'Peace'."

Despite an outbreak of summer diarrhoea, the atmosphere almost of euphoria continued, St. Quentin noting that a man named Brown, who had been transferred from the County Prison as an ungovernable lunatic, was sitting "as quiet as a child eating a crust of bread" and later that 22 of the male patients "were gone to work at digging potatoes for Mr. Stevington – this I consider to be a most satisfactory arrangement". Another of the visitors was agreeably surprised to see the quality of the work done by the female patients: ". . . I hope every assistance will be given to the sale of them".

As the winter of 1856/7 approached many of the original installations were giving trouble, but the justices were understandably reluctant to incur much expenditure on replacements in view of the imminence of the building of the Three Counties Asylum.* When the scullery boiler became overheated and burst, permission was sought from Mr. Stuart, the visiting magistrate for the month, to replace it with a new boiler made of iron; this, it was suggested, would probably cost no more than what they could get from the sale of the old copper. The new one was installed only five days later, but Stuart was cautious in his response to the suggestion that it be fitted with a ballcock and cistern to reduce the danger of its bursting also: "As this would increase the expense by about 3£ *[sic]* I directed them to wait till the meeting of the committee. The iron boiler will cost about 16s. and the old copper sold for 24s. leaving a balance in our favour of 8s."

The case of James Wallace, deceased:

The Commissioners in Lunacy, or their staff, were always quick to pounce on irregularities in documentation that might indicate possible malpractice in the handling of patients. James Wallace, a patient at the Bedford asylum, had been sent home on two months' trial by John Harris shortly before Denne's arrival.

On December 14th 1854 a scribbled note was received by Samuel Wing:

* Now Fairfield Hospital, itself due for ultimate closure and care of the remaining patients "in the community".

"J. Wallace
Dear Sir,
This man is dead – I will *[illegible]* & send you a certificate
Yrs faithfully
Geo Girby Ware"

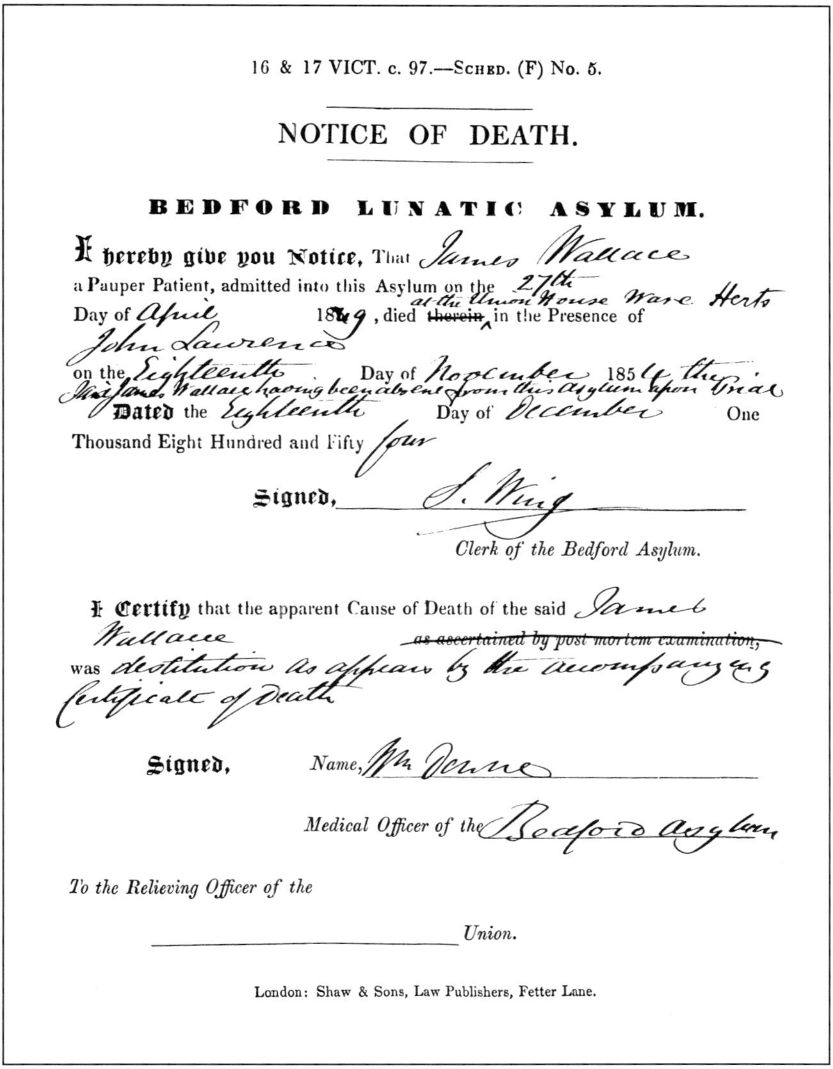

16 & 17 VICT. c. 97.—SCHED. (F) No. 5.

NOTICE OF DEATH.

BEDFORD LUNATIC ASYLUM.

I hereby give you Notice, That James Wallace a Pauper Patient, admitted into this Asylum on the 27th Day of April 1849, died ~~therein~~ at the Union House Ware Herts in the Presence of John Lawrence on the Eighteenth Day of November 1854 the said James Wallace having been absent from this Asylum upon Trial
Dated the Eighteenth Day of December One Thousand Eight Hundred and Fifty four

Signed, J. Wing
Clerk of the Bedford Asylum.

I Certify that the apparent Cause of Death of the said James Wallace ~~as ascertained by post mortem examination,~~ was destitution as appears by the accompanying Certificate of Death

Signed, *Name,* Wm Denne

Medical Officer of the Bedford Asylum

To the Relieving Officer of the
_______________ *Union.*

London: Shaw & Sons, Law Publishers, Fetter Lane.

The commissioners wrote to Wing on December 23rd – when did Wallace leave the asylum? What provision had been made for his care and maintenance? And other particulars were requested: "The Board consider the case as one calling for serious enquiry." The matter was investigated: the discharge on two months' trial had been on Harris's advice; as nothing had been heard at the expiry of the time Samuel Wing had written to the Ware Union saying that detention in an asylum was no longer necessary. In reply, he had been informed that James Wallace had died in the workhouse there.

The Commissioners asked for a death certificate and William Denne obligingly provided one, stating the cause of death as "destitution".

John Harris wrote on December 26th from Springfield House:

> "James Wallace was quiet and harmless. he was constantly employed in the gardens and had frequently entreated me to allow him to go home. I thought he could be taken care of in the Union House [the workhouse] as well as in the asylum."

From the Ware Union, December 27th:

> Wallace had been allowed by their Board of Guardians two shillings a week [as outdoor relief] and when he asked for more the allowance was increased to three shillings, which he continued to receive up to the time of his death. "That was sufficient for his maintenance, taken with what he was able to earn."
>
> On hearing that he was ill "the Relieving Officer went to see him and finding that he could not receive that care and attention at his lodgings which his condition seemed to demand, caused him to be removed to the Union Workhouse". Wallace died two days later, having been ill "but a very short time before he was taken into the House". Originally the guardians had wanted him to stay in the Union but as he had objected the Board felt that they couldn't insist – he had been discharged on trial from the asylum and had been provided with outdoor relief. . . .

CHAPTER TEN

Endgames: 1856-60

The annual visit by the Commissioners in Lunacy was conducted by R. M. Lutteridge and J. Wilkes on December 12th 1856, and their report and recommendations present a vivid picture of the state of the asylum in its closing stages.

Since the last visit in July 1855 there had been 153 admissions and 76 discharges; of the latter, 56 had recovered. There had been 60 deaths which had been ascribed to the following causes:

Pulmonary disease	10
Paralysis	12
Epilepsy	9
General debility	8
Dysentery and diarrhoea	7
Apoplexy [stroke]	3
Dropsy [swollen limbs etc.]	1
Erysipelas [skin infection]	1
Exhaustion after mania	4
Heart disease	2
Natural decay [old age]	1
Marasmus [malnutrition]	1
Suffocation during epileptic fit	1

No cases of suicide had occurred in the period (Elizabeth Biggs had died a month before the previous visit, and the storeman, John Howes, was a member of the staff, albeit for only a few days). Nevertheless, the commissioners recommended removal of the iron bars over the doors of the sleeping rooms as they afforded "facilities for suicide".

The total number of patients was 313, of whom 152 were male and 161 female. Three patients were absent on trial at home. All the patients were seen except for one woman who had been admitted a few days before, in a feeble condition and in a maniacal state.

In the medical case-book it was recorded that on admission:

> "... she was tightly bound in a strait jacket, covered with bruises and having also a large wound on the left shinbone. her wrists and ankles bore marks of ligatures which had produced ulceration."

Over 200 of the patients were employed in various ways; of the 81 men, 35 worked outdoors as labourers and nine as artisans. One hundred and twenty-three women were occupied, 45 in needlework, 13 in plaiting straw and 28 in the washhouse and laundry.

> "We are informed that during the last six months, bonnets and clothing have been made by the female patients for sale to the poor at low, but remunerative rates."

Prayers were read daily in the chapel, and on Sundays, divine service was performed by the chaplain; about 60 patients of each sex attended. It was recommended that patients should be given "a better description of dress for Sundays".

Some points made in the previous report were picked up. All the tailoring and shoe-making work was now done at the asylum. There was a fairly good supply of "amusing books", and some prints were being framed to be hung in the day-rooms.

One of the walls had been *slightly* lowered and all the windows were now free from wire-work except for certain sleeping quarters. A regular night watch had been introduced on each side. However, the commissioners felt that a better kind of bedding should be provided for sick or bed-ridden patients. "Horsehair or wool should in *all* cases be substituted for chaff in the pillows."

They had been informed that the new asylum would not be built for three or four years yet and therefore urged on the committee of visiting justices the need to make every provision for the comfort and well-being of the patients (such provision not involving, however, any great outlay on structural alterations). The asylum was badly overcrowded, and as the justices had ruled out the renting of extra accommodation, the commissioners favoured an increase in the number of home trials. The Lunatic Asylums Act of 1853 (Section 79) had, they pointed out, encouraged the boarding out of harmless and incurable patients who "with the aid of an adequate weekly allowance may be properly taken care of by their friends".

The report concluded with words of praise:

> "Having regard to the disadvantages under which the institution now labours, both from its overcrowded state and structural imperfections, we think that its management and condition reflect much credit upon the medical superintendent [Denne], matron [Mrs. Denne] and other officers."

The Christmas festivities of 1856, for which the patients prepared the decorations "cheerfully and remarkably free from excitement", were somewhat marred by a piece of attempted chicanery by a local contractor. In the light of the adverse remarks about the bedding, some more blankets had been ordered for the asylum. The two justices on duty, William Stuart Jr. and Lynn Smart, were asked to look at some samples that had been submitted by a Mr. Sturges. The blankets "... came in a wet state having evidently been dampened to increase the weight. We decided to refuse the whole tender [which was for other goods as well] without inspection".

Provision of a new padded room had been agreed but its construction was delayed for some months because supplies of coir fibre were still awaited. The room was eventually ready by April and was used thereafter mainly for those epileptics who tended to injure themselves by falling out of bed.

By the summer of 1857, the building of the Three Counties Asylum had already begun and the commissioners, B. W. Procter and James Wilkes, said that ". . . we forbear from making several suggestions which occur to us, from the very imperfect structure of the present establishment".* However, there were some suggestions unrelated to the building itself which would not be expensive to implement:

The female wing was badly infested with bedbugs and W. H. Whitbread and T. C. Higgins had reported in May "some part of the house in confusion owing to the turning out of the beds in No. 3 gallery, female side, on account of the alarming increase of bugs". The commissioners advised that the wooden partitions which

---

* The Bedford General Infirmary, on the other side of Ampthill road, and which had been built in 1803, had to wait for a further 30 years before the many deficiencies in its fabric were to receive attention – see *Private Charity and the Public Purse.*

formed very small single rooms be removed ("swept away" was the rather more decisive term employed). The old wooden bedsteads ought to be removed and, as a gesture to thrift, some of them might be used to make sunshades and seats in the grounds. Iron bedsteads should be provided; they could be taken to the new asylum in due course.

The suggestions were adopted by the following spring and extended on the advice of Lynn Smart and W. B. Higgins; the wainscotting and doors of the galleries were to be divided into lots and sold by private contract at valuation by a Mr. Conquest, a Kempston builder. The ultimate fate of this material and whatever livestock it still contained is unknown, but for the asylum, Captain Wm. Stuart Jnr. thought that "... the wards made by throwing down the partitions are a great improvement and they are far better than Barrack Rooms".

At the time of the commissioners' visit the number of inmates had reached a record total – **323**. In the previous 18 months there had been 48 new admissions, 12 discharged and 12 deaths (mainly from general paralysis, a complication of syphilis).

It was, they considered, "impracticable for only one medical gentleman to superintend and manage an asylum of this size without assistance". (In the absence of any evidence to the contrary, it has to be assumed either that there was no house surgeon in post at the time or that the commissioners did not consider his duties as being part of the superintendence or management. In any case, it is interesting to note that they appear to have drawn a distinction between these two functions.)

In view of the overcrowding more patients should be sent out on leave and some chronic cases remitted to workhouses. In their view, three shillings and sixpence a week was an inadequate allowance for patients on leave. Pressure on all licensed (private) houses and most other asylums was so great at that time that there was, in their view, no possibility of transferring patients to other institutions.

The suggestion that more patients be sent out on home leave was acted upon, and in many cases the justices depended on the parish surgeons or other medical men to advise on the patients' suitability for continuing care "in the community". Sometimes, however, they preferred to rely on their own judgment, as was the case with Jane Hutton.

Thomas Trew, surgeon, of Aspley Guise certified that he had personally examined Jane Hutton, a patient absent on trial in her home and:

> ". . . that he found as to her state of mind she states that God's angels have fed her on and off for 20 years and that she is much annoyed by people under the bricks of the floor who throw stones at her, otherwise she is quiet and harmless but talks and mumbles to herself, and that her detention in an asylum is no longer necessary."

The committee did not agree that she was fit to be at large . . . "having taken into consideration the delusions under which the patient still labours" and they directed her to be retaken and brought back to the asylum.

A funeral party: At about three-thirty one afternoon in August, William St. Quentin arrived to find "a party of female mourners" assembled at the entrance in great trouble at having been too late to attend the funeral of a female relative who had died in the asylum. The funeral, according to William Denne and the Rev. Mr. Swann, had been arranged for two o'clock at their particular request, but they maintained that the only notice that they had received was that it was to take place at half-past three. It seemed that their particular concern was less at having missed the opportunity to express their grief at the ceremony than to secure a small book belonging to the deceased; what it contained was not stated.

A search for the book was undertaken without success and it was presumed that their late relative, who was said to be "of a violent and destructive character" had destroyed it.

St. Quentin wisely left them to continue the discussion with the medical superintendent and went on his way in the company of the assistant matron and Barnes, the steward.

The coroner, Mr. E. Eagles, reported to the justices in October that an inquest had been held on a patient named John Sage, and that the jury verdict was that he had "died from suffocation caused by strangulation inflicted by himself, being at the time of his death 34 years old". Captain Stuart made the rather oddly-phrased comment that "although he was of a suicidal nature he had given no indication to suppose he meditated any act of this kind".

April 27th 1858 (William Bartholomew Higgins):

> "There was a sudden addition to the inmates of this asylum by the delivery of Mary Gray of a fine boy at 11 o'clock last night. Mother and child are doing well."

July 15th: George Hurst, then vice-chairman of the Bedford Union and three others visited as a committee of the Board of Guardians. There were 30 patients belonging to the Bedford Union and:

> ". . . we cannot express too highly the satisfaction we experienced at the judicious treatment and the humane attention received by the unfortunate inmates of the establishment . . . everything is done to restore all cases to society which are by human means susceptible of improvement."

George Hurst was an outstanding figure of the Bedford scene for many years.* Born in 1800, he became a successful draper in the town and played a prominent part in the affairs of the Bedford Union and in the Borough. He was five times mayor of Bedford and died just before his 99th birthday. Alderman Hurst had paid an official visit to the asylum the previous year as a member of the committee, which had been appointed to keep an eye on the pauper lunatics sent in from the Borough, under the provisions of the Lunatic Asylums Act of 1853.

The case of Ruth Pedder: The Rev. C. C. Beaty Pownall visited and was taken round by Barnes, the steward and the deputy matron. Denne and his wife were "enjoying a three-weeks relaxation from their labours". While engaged in writing his report, Mr. Beaty Pownall was told that a female patient named Ruth Pedder, who was in seclusion, had hanged herself:

> ". . . on going round the female side with the deputy matron I passed the door of the cell in which the poor creature was & heard her talking loudly & moving about restlessly – but did not see her (the only case I believe in which I failed to see a patient) nor have the door opened, as the deputy matron said that she

---

* See *Private Charity and the Public Purse*, p. 13.

> was very unquiet & thought my presence would add to her excitement. The fatal act must have been committed immediately after our quitting the gallery. Mr. Johnson the house surgeon of the Infirmary was at once sent for & attended with the utmost promptness . . . after he had seen the body he stated that she was quite dead, beyond any hope of resuscitation. She had twisted the sheet round her neck and suspended herself to the bars of the window. . . ."

An inquest was held on the following day with the customary verdict. Ruth Pedder was 35 years old at the time of her death.

A few days later, Henry Littledale noted:

> "The interment of the poor woman who committed suicide and on whose case the coroner has reported . . . is postponed till Sunday next to enable the husband, a very poor man, to give his attendance."

Another potentially suicidal patient, Elizabeth Disher, required constant attention day and night which was, Beaty-Pownall wrote, the more inconvenient because of the continued illness of "the female attendant Ball", who was reported by John Harris to be in great danger – she was suffering from dysentery. Mr. and Mrs. Denne were still on leave – "Mr. Harris kindly visits the establishment twice a day".

By July 30th, both the patient and the attendant were better despite fears that the latter wouldn't survive, and when Littledale visited on August 3rd, the patient appeared "tranquil", but nevertheless he "cautioned the servants . . . to be extremely vigilant and they appear to be taking all the precuations possible".

December 24th 1858: (Thomas Charles Higgins)

> "I found the patients in the house all cheerful and happy. I was gratified at observing the interest taken by them in the formation of the Xmas devices of evergreen – wherein much taste is evinced both as regards the mottos and designs . . . the patients are to have roast beef and plum pudding tomorrow, and in a few days hence there is to be a Xmas tree."

During 1859, in the closing stages before the transfer, there was little for the visitors to report. Wm. Lynn Smart (Bedfordshire) went round with Marlborough Pryor (Hertfordshire) in June, they having been appointed by the newly constituted committee of visitors of the Three Counties asylum.

". . . to make a selection of such articles in the institution as are deemed proper to be transferred to the new asylum when it is located." They made out a list of suitable furniture, bedding, kitchen utensils etc.

On June 29th, Henry Littledale was alarmed to find one of the patients, Henry Palmer, in "what appeared to me a frightful state of fits". Denne was away and the Infirmary had been asked to assist. Unfortunately, Johnson, the house surgeon there, was also absent and ". . . a youth had come and I saw him [the patient] again – but not being satisfied, I had Mr. Harris sent for & he came while I was here & found the man's alarming state from congestion of the brain . . .". Palmer died at 4.30 the following morning.

Littledale recorded the fact that the patient's friends removed the body to "his place of abode" in Hertfordshire and were "well satisfied that every thing needful had been done for him".

The last visit by the commissioners to the Bedford asylum took place on December 22nd 1859. It was made by Messrs. Lutteridge and Gaskell:

Since the previous year there had been 135 admissions, 85 discharges (59 of whom had recovered) and 49 deaths. With one exception (suicide) the causes of death were of an ordinary kind – general paralysis, epilepsy and general debility. They were particularly impressed by "the tranquil and contented aspect of the worst class of male patients".

The average number of patients engaged in some useful kind of employment was 165; 80 men and 85 women. There was room in the chapel for 100 people and it was full every Sunday. From 12 to 20 male patients went out beyond the bounds of the asylum every Sunday afternoon ". . . and about 25 of each sex are taken out for recreation to regattas etc. The female patients occupied in the laundry department walk out on Saturday afternoons to the number of 20 or 30".

"Taking into consideration the shortness of the period during which the patients will continue to reside in the present asylum, from whence, we are given to understand, they will be transferred to the new asylum near Hitchin about February next, we abstain from recommending any outlay upon structural improvements or a further supply, much needed, of comfortable furniture. . . . For the same reason we do not now suggest the laying out and planting of the airing courts which being only gravelled, have a cheerless aspect."

William Denne was commended for his active exertions in preparing for the move. His enthusiasm for the task had no doubt been enhanced by his appointment as the first medical superintendent of the Three Counties Asylum (and that of Mrs. Denne to the post of matron) and he was to remain there for the next 14 years. A casual visitor to Bedford in 1857, I. L. Levison, of Dorset Square, London, could not:

". . . but express my admiration of this noble institution; and of the professional and psycological *[sic]* qualifications of Mr. Denne for his philanthropy, talent and excellent tact in the management of a class of patients, whose cerebral organisation, in the majority of the cases, are of a low character: which, superadded to a nearly general deficiency of all systematic and moral and intellectual training and many having injured themselves by animal excesses, renders the task of surveillance on the part of this medical gentleman so much more difficult and more onerous. And, hence, the great satisfaction I have experienced."

By the summer of 1859, the building of the new asylum was well under way and in July the chaplain, the Rev. Edward Swann, reported the results of a consumer survey:

"A party of ten patients were taken this week to view the New Asylum ar Arlesey. They were highly delighted. Several of them have told me their opinions of the chapel and the new arrangements. Some seem to think it will be a most complete and cheerful residence – one woman told me she thought the effect upon the patients would be most salutory; another said it would be very dull, there would be no society for it was a long way from any town."

In September 1859 it was decided that all books and papers relating to the patients then in detention would be sent to the new asylum; all others relating to the county of Bedford were to go to the muniment room in the town. "Useless" documents and bills were to be destroyed (after the committee had reviewed them). Notice was to be given to all officers that their duties would be terminated by the following Lady Day. This brought from the visiting surgeon, John Harris, the following plea:

> "December 12th 1859:
>
> Gentlemen,
>
> In consequence of a notice I received from the Committee of Visitors of the Three Counties Lunatic Asylum at Arlesey – that my services would not be required at the old asylum after Lady Day next, I applied to them to reinstate me in the same position as I held in the old one in conformity of a resolution passed by your committee on the 8th. day of August 1854 when on the faith of that resolution I resigned my appointment.
>
> Having received no intimation that the Committee of Visitors at Arlesey had entertained my request I have now to place my case in your hands fully trusting that you will see me righted.
>
> J. Harris."

In the event, the committee of visitors to the new asylum (which included a contingent from Bedfordshire) decided against the appointment of a visiting surgeon, and John Harris, with the support of W. H. Whitbread and Henry Littledale, pressed his claim to a pension – to which he was fully entitled under the terms of his appointment in Bedford. The matter was raised at the court of quarter sessions in October 1860 and gave rise to lively discussion.

The claim, said Mr. Whitbread, was a just one and the county was in any case bound to pay Mr. Harris £50 per annum; he had served the county faithfully and honestly for over 30 years. The proposed allowance was inadequate and he would move "in round numbers" that it be increased to £100 – the other counties were, he considered, in honour bound to pay their share; they were parties to the original agreement. Henry Littledale spoke to the same effect.

After some discussion the chairman, T. C. Higgins, said that the county couldn't possibly be called upon to pay more than £50 –

"Mr. Harris never dreamt of such a thing. The court had no power in the matter, nor was there any fund from which any further allowance could be paid."

He didn't often intrude his opinion upon the court, he said, but when any suggestion was made of an illegal character he felt bound to interfere. He had a sincere regard for Mr. Harris and if he could wink at any little irregularity he would do so in his case.

It was agreed that the question of Harris's pension (his "memorial") would be referred to the other counties involved in the hope that they would see the justice of carrying out the promise that had been made to him.

Alas, not only did the other counties refuse to contribute their fair share, but the agreed pension of £50 per annum couldn't legally be paid either from the county rate or from the old asylum fund, which was now closed. After lengthy discussion at the court of quarter sessions in January 1860, the subject was finally dropped.

John Harris died at his home in Kempston on July 2nd 1861. He was 58 years old at the time of his death, which received public notice only in a report in the *Bedfordshire Times* of a meeting of the governors of the Bedford General Infirmary (where the young Harris had been house surgeon):

> "The Rev. J. T. Day said they had been doing honour to the memory of a great man. [The Duke of Bedford had just died and the governors had resolved on a memorial to him; it took the form of a portrait which is still to be seen at the South Wing of Bedford Hospital.] Now, said Mr. Day, perhaps they would not object to pay a tribute to the memory of one who occupied a humbler position, but one who had been . . . sincerely respected by all who knew him – he alluded to the late Mr. Harris, of Springfield."

A letter of condolence was sent to the family on the governors' behalf.

Four of the existing senior staff at Bedford were appointed to the new asylum; they were the medical superintendent, William Denne (whose salary at Bedford was £200 p.a.), the matron, Lucy Denne (£100), John Barnes, the steward (£80), and Samuel Wing, clerk to the visiting justices (£100).

Edward Swann, the chaplain (£100 per annum), had hoped to obtain the corresponding post at Arlesey, and when it was advertised in October 1859, he wrote as instructed for further particulars, only to receive the standard reply, which in draft form read:

> "In answer to your enquiries, two full services on the Sunday, morning prayers in the week days and daily visits to the patients, as well as performing the burial service over those who die in the asylum.
>
> I enclose a list of the Visitors but personal canvassing will not be countenanced. The house will be about half a mile from the asylum and is situated near the Great Northern Railway."

Marlborough Pryor, chairman of the new committee, wrote to Thomas Charles Higgins on October 30th 1859 to say that there were 80 candidates already for the chaplaincy ". . . when your clerk has a little leisure I should be glad of the list giving simply the names and residences". He added: "I do not think that Mr. Swann has any cause for complaint for we never proposed to transfer the officers from one asylum to the other."

The existing committee of visiting magistrates continued to serve in that capacity for the new asylum until 1861. Meetings were held at Arlesey and special arrangements were made for those members travelling from Bedford:

From Samuel Wing to Seymour Clarke Esq., General Manager, Great Northern Railway, Kings Cross Station, November 21st 1859:

> "Dear Sir, Our next general meeting of the Committee of Visitors of the asylum near Arlesey is on Monday 28th. inst. Will you please direct the usual trains to stop at the siding?"

Notice was given in the local press concerning the new asylum, which would be opened for the reception of pauper lunatics from the counties of Bedford, Hertford and Huntingdon from April 2nd, 1860. No patients would be admitted to the Bedford asylum after March 29th.

Printed notices of the arrangements which had been made with the Great Northern Railway for certain trains to stop at Arlesey station on weekdays could be obtained by application to the asylum or to the committee of visitors in St. Cuthbert Street.

The first batch of 100 patients was transferred by rail to the

THREE COUNTIES ASYLUM,

NEAR ARLESEY, BEDFORDSHIRE.

The Committee of Visitors have arranged with the Great Northern Railway Company that from

MARCH 1st, UNTIL FURTHER NOTICE,

the following Trains will be stopped at the Asylum Platform, *on a Signal being given there*, or *on request from parties travelling by them*, at Arlesey or Hitchin, as the case may be, viz.—

DOWN.				UP.			
	1	2	3		1	2	3
	A. M.	P. M.	P. M.		A. M.	A. M.	P. M.
LONDON	10. 5	1 .45	5 . 5	ARLESEY	7 .52	11 .30	3 .45
ARLESEY	11 .36	3 . 0	6 .24	LONDON	9 .30	1 . 0	5 .30

The Arlesey Fares to be charged to and from the Asylum Platform.

March 1*st*, 1860.

asylum at Arlesey in February 1860, leaving 208 awaiting removal; that was effected in succeeding weeks, and by early April, the task – no mean one – was complete. It might be thought that such events would have captured the imagination of the local journalists, but no mention appeared in the press. That was possibly because they were preoccupied by the notorious trial (and later public execution at Bedford prison*) of Joseph Castle, the Luton wife-murderer. Alternatively, the justices may have taken care to keep the physical transfer of such large groups of mentally disturbed patients out of the public appetite for drama; that would have been adequately met already.

Although details of the rail transfer are lacking, one indication of its difficulties may be gleaned from the warm commendation given to William Denne by the justices at the midsummer quarter sessions

* The *Bedfordshire Times* reporter, in close attendance at the hanging, wrote that there had been a heavy downpour of rain beforehand, and that the wood of the scaffold had swollen. When the bolt was withdrawn, the trap failed to open: "... this was at once remedied." The reporter said that the condemned man, "being earnestly engaged in prayer . . . must have been unconscious of any delay, nor was he subjected to the slightest inconvenience". (!)

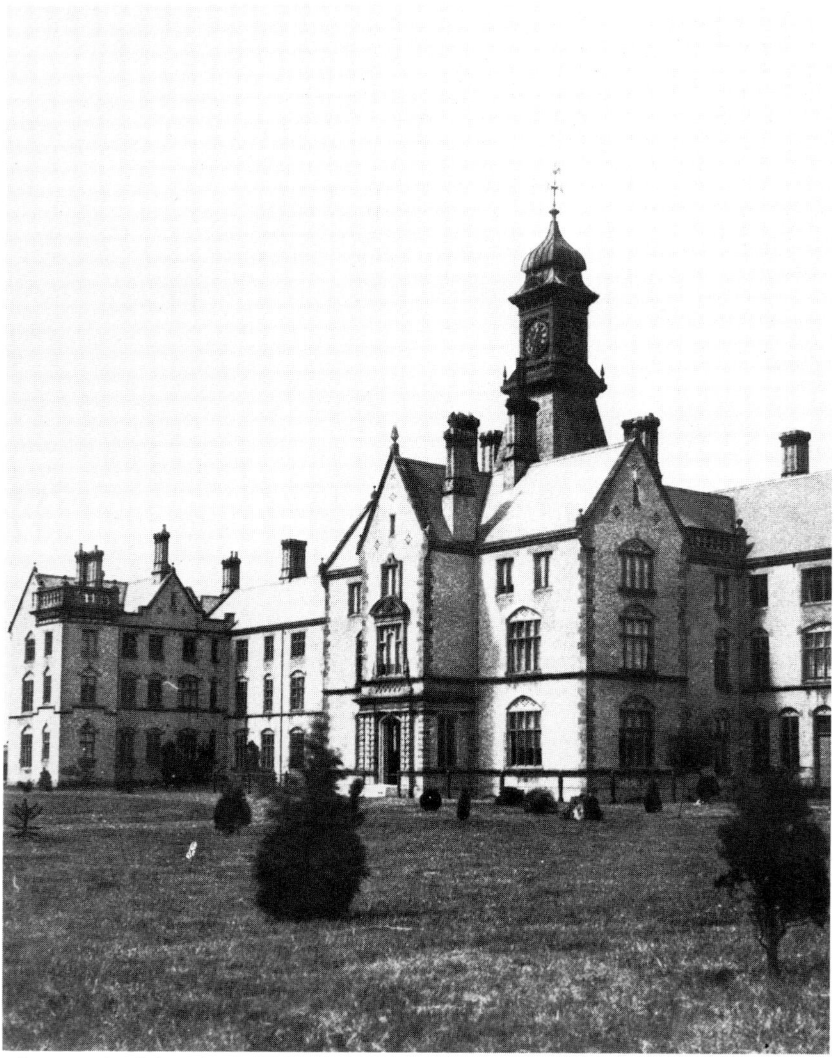

Photograph of the Three Counties asylum (1870). From a series of paper negatives by the architect, G.F. Jones. County Record Office

for "the masterly way in which he had produced order and regularity from a state of chaos". There was also the report the following January by the visiting justices to the new asylum that there had been 37 deaths since it opened in April: "... the number is large but it is caused most probably by the excitement consequent upon the removal."

That was by no means the end of the story of their asylum for the Bedford magistrates, however. They still had to balance the accounts and above all, to dispose of the building, its contents and the land on which it stood.

A notice had been placed in the local newspapers in March 1860:

"Bedfordshire Lunatic Asylum.

> The Committee of Visitors request that all persons to whom they are indebted in respect of this Institution will forward particulars of their claims to the asylum by or before ten o'clock on the morning of Monday, the 26th. day of March instant, to enable the committee to close their accounts preparatory to the asylum being given up."

It was reported at the court of quarter sessions in July 1860 that: ". . . the balance on loan of the old asylum will be £1,095 after payment of instalment and interest of £401.10s. The committee would desire to recommend that the balance be discharged whenever a sale can be effected of the asylum's estate." Previously, claims had been settled out of the asylum revenues, but as these had now ceased, the county rate would have to bear the charge.

This brought a swift reaction from Mr. R. L. Orlebar, according to the account of the meeting in the *Bedfordshire Times*:

> "With regard to the lunatic asylum the magistrates [had] thought it their duty to carry out an improved scheme for the treatment of lunatics and had built a very good and a very large establishment. He had originally objected to the scheme but the other day thought it his duty to visit the new asylum and was on the whole very pleased with what he saw. The old asylum would have done for this county but the justices wanted to bring in the other two counties.
>
> Now they wanted to sell the old one it probably wouldn't bring in more than one tenth of what it [had] cost."

(It seems that John Harvey – of Ickwell Bury – did not voice his own reservations at the time, but he was to take a leading part in certain recriminations that followed at later meetings; he had resigned from the building committee of the Three Counties asylum ostensibly because he was going to be abroad for some time.)

The chairman of quarter sessions, Thomas Charles Higgins (ever the diplomat), reported that now that the works had been completed and the building occupied, the visitors had thought it right to invite the magistrates to pay a visit. A large number had attended, he said, and had expressed their complete satisfaction.

The fears expressed by Mr. Orlebar and others about the likely difficulties of disposing of the old asylum proved to be fully justified, and the following account of the transactions in which the justices became involved will provide, perhaps, a suitable epilogue to the story of the Bedford lunatic asylum.

CHAPTER ELEVEN

Epilogue: the last accounts

Six months before it closed, the justices had turned their attention to the important question of what was to happen to the Bedford asylum when the patients had all been transferred to the Three Counties. They decided that the building with its contents and the land on which it stood was to be sold off and in September 1859 an advertisement was placed for four successive weeks – in the *London Times, Builder, Leeds Intelligence, Midland Counties Herald, Manchester Guardian* and other national papers as well as in the two county newspapers of the day – the *Bedfordshire Times* and the *Bedford Mercury*:

> "To managers of public institutions, manufacturers and other capitalists:
>
> For sale, the Bedford County Lunatic Asylum about to be given up in consequence of the erection of a new asylum. The Bedford asylum consists of a centre building 166 feet in length, of a most substantial character of brick, with stone quoins and string courses and double-revealed circular head sashes: the greater part of the timber is of oak. The residence in the centre comprises a commodious dwelling with suitable kitchen and offices. On each side of the centre building are wings of two stories about 230 feet in length together with washhouses and laundries about 80 feet in length
>
> The airing courts are enclosed with about 1200 feet of sound brick walling 10 feet in height, attached are farm buildings, piggeries and workshops. The property consists altogether of $9^{a}.2^{r}.12^{p}$ and is bounded on the west by the turnpike road leading from Bedford to Woburn, on the east by the Bletchley branch of the London & North Western Railway (from which the property is divided by a substantial brick wall) and on the north and south by land the property of His Grace the Duke of Bedford and is distant from Bedford less than a mile. The

> Midland Railway is in the immediate proximity of the asylum. There is a good supply of pure water.
>
> The land is freehold, land tax redeemed, and tithe-free gas is laid on to the asylum. The premises may be viewed upon application to the Resident Medical Officer . . . possession can be given on 5th. April 1860."

Understandably, perhaps, there was no mention of a report made the previous month by the Inspector of Nuisances of Bedford Town. It stated (in terms suited to the legal minds at which it was directed), that "the public water course at the back of the asylum into which the asylum drains run is in a foul and offensive state owing to the asylum drainage". The justices ordered that the drain be cleaned out.

The response to the advertisement offering the asylum for sale was, as might have been expected, disappointing. A Canadian, the Rev. A. Lendrum of St. Margaret's College, Crieff, N.B., made an offer to buy it, and his letter was accompanied by one from a London architect which indicated that (presumably on his advice) Mr. Lendrum was prepared to pay a maximum of £5,000. The committee were "not inclined to entertain the application"; in any case, when Lendrum later inspected the premises he withdrew his offer, on the grounds that the cost of alterations would be too great for his purpose (whatever that was). Similarly, an offer of £3,650 by James Tacy Wing and George Hurst was unacceptably low.

Looking ahead to the time when outstanding claims would no longer be settled out of the asylum revenues, but would fall directly on the county rates, the visiting justices decided to call in the experts. The chairman, Thomas Charles Higgins, was empowered to engage the London firm of Farebrother, Clarke and Lye to advise them on the sale. A selection from the ensuing correspondence follows:

November 9th 1859: (Mr. Higgins to Messrs Farebrother & Co.):

Enclosed were samples of the advertisement which had been placed in various journals which would explain that the visiting justices were desirous of selling the asylum. No acceptable tenders had been received and ". . . the visitors think you might be able from your experience to offer them useful advice". The chairman invited them to attend the meeting of the committee to be held on Tuesday December 13th. On what terms, he asked, would they come to

Bedford to look over the property, to advise on the best way of disposing of it and on the amount it could be expected to yield? If all else failed, might it be advisable to sell the asylum by auction?

November 12th.: (Messrs. Farebrother & Co. to Mr. Higgins):

They apologised for what they called their failure to reply fully earlier as the partners were absent. They would be happy to attend at Bedford on Tuesday 15th. instant to advise on disposal and valuation etc. Their fee would be 20 guineas *exclusive of travelling expenses.*

> ". . . We have much to do with this class of property having sold some years since the Government Prison at Dartmoor, all the Metropolitan Police Stations and more recently the House of Correction and County Gaol at Guildford, Surrey, of which we forward you particulars of the sale, showing the mode in which they were sold and the sums they realised. . . ."

November 14th.: (Mr. Higgins to Messrs. Farebrother & Co.):

> "I am not authorized to offer you a larger sum than 20 guineas for your visit to the asylum on the 15th. prox° what was meant to include all expenses. Your visit therefore must be postponed till after the 15th . . . or you must consent to come on the 15th. subject to the decision of the Visiting Justices in relation to the travelling expenses – I may add that a return ticket from London to Bedford and back is 12/8ᵈ. You may be at Bedford from Kings Cross at 8.48 or at 10.44. . . . Pray let me hear again from you."

November 15th.: Messrs. Farebrother & Co. to Mr. Higgins:

> "We have to acknowledge your favour of the 14th. current and are perfectly willing to include the Bagatelle you mention, but it appeared to us to be one of those matters wherein we ought, in advising the Magistrates, to come down the day before when many points might suggest themselves which a hurried and cursory visit would fail to supply.
>
> In your favour of yesterday you say the 15th. prox° and repeat it a second time, by which we assume the 15th. to be the day, though your letter of the 9th. says Tuesday 13th. – Be pleased to advise us hereon as also the hour of meeting. . . ."

November 16th.: (Mr. Higgins to Messrs. Farebrother & Co.):

> "Gentlemen – The monthly meeting of the Visitors at the Bedford Asylum is on Tuesday 13th. prox° and not on the 15th. as I in error said in my last – We meet at one o'clock, so that you would have two or three hours before that time to make a survey of the premises. . . ."

Mr. Clarke, of Messrs. Farebrother, Clarke and Lye duly travelled to Bedford (at the firm's own expense) on December 13th. and his report followed a week later; whether the magistrates considered that they had obtained good value for their money was never recorded:

> "The questions submitted for our consideration were first, as to the best mode of disposing of the asylum and secondly as to the sum it ought to yield on a sale.
>
> As to the first, the course which we are informed you have adopted viz. advertizing in the London and local papers is the best, and should be continued because with an important property designed expressly for one object and applicable to but comparatively few others, a much longer period will probably have to be taken in finding a purchaser, and forcing the property into the public market would, if there were no such building and premises required at that particular period, tend to diminish the value.
>
> Delay, in our judgement, will be the means of obtaining the best price as it not infrequently happens that when peculiar or class property has been for some time before the public it may suggest itself to the government and others: 'Why, here are the particular premises adapted to our purposes.'*
>
> In this case, and in reply to your second question we believe a sum of £10,000 might be obtained but as a mere speculation it might realise between 5 and 6,000; and in the last alternative a forced sale of the materials and afterwards the land, and we are of opinion they would realise together barely £5,000 and we have very grave doubts whether such a large quantity of materials, especially bricks, could be sold at any one time in the town of Bedford, and the expense would of course be materially increased."

---

* Just how frequently governments have ever recognised such serendipity seems doubtful!

An approach to the government as a possible buyer of the asylum had already been tried and the justices had received a dusty answer:

> November 1859: Samuel Wing to the Quartermaster General: "Sir, The committee of visitors of the County Lunatic Asylum at Bedford will feel obliged if you will do them the favor of granting a personal interview to one of their body for the purpose of again bringing under your notice the desirability of the purchase of this property by the government for some military purpose as they would be unwilling to dispose of the property in question without giving the War Department an opportunity of considering this proposal. . . ."

> December 5th.: The Quartermaster General to Samuel Wing: "Sir, In answer to your letters dated 15th. ultimo and the 3rd. instant . . . respecting a personal interview with a gentleman deputed to urge the purchase of the Bedford Lunatic Asylum and property attached thereto – I beg to inform you that having been in communication with the authorities of the War Office upon the subject I find that the question of adapting this building to Barrack purposes was fully gone into four years ago and that it was then decided after mature consideration that it was not desirable to treat with the local authorities for the acquisition of the property. . . . Ready as I am to receive the gentleman deputed by the committee to visit me I regret that I am not prepared to advise him to come to London for that purpose."

In May 1860, an inventory of the furniture, fittings and fixtures, was approved for sale by auction, with the exception of a few items destined for the new asylum. The sale took place on June 25th. and 26th. and realised the sum of £423.15s.3d.

The Three Counties asylum had been designed by George Fowler Jones, the York architect who had accompanied Samuel Hill on the survey of the Bedford establishment that they had conducted eight years before [see p. 105]. The justices learned that the total cost of the new institution amounted to £115,000. The successful tender for the building works had been submitted by a Mr. Webster of Boston (Lincs.) in the sum of £53,626. These figures produced from John Harvey the first rumblings of the discontent which had caused his resignation from the building committee earlier.

Mr. Harvey had not intended to say anything about the asylum, he insisted, although he had felt deeply on the subject; ". . . no good object can be obtained by making up old stories". He had felt it his duty to have protested in writing about the proceedings of the building committee and he didn't wish to say anything against them now: "they had built us the very best lunatic asylum in England, in Europe [and], he believed, in the world" – but it should be understood that "the plan was not his plan and he protested against being in any way held responsible for the enormous, and in his opinion, unnecessary expense which had been incurred by the committee".

By April 1861 the building had still not been sold and it was agreed to advertise again. The chairman drew attention to the fact that a considerable sum had already been spent in advertising and the committee thought that it might be worthwhile offering the building for lease instead. William Denne had heard from someone who "had some idea of hiring the old asylum", and some particulars following the letter had suggested that it might be suitable as a *branch* asylum for pauper lunatics.

The chairman, T. C. Higgins, confirmed that "the number of pauper lunatics was increasing at an enormous rate and it might be necessary for us to increase the accommodation for our own lunatics".

(This was a remarkable thought, under the circumstances. A "branch" asylum in Bedford would have been treated as a separate establishment with its own staff, committee of visiting justices and above all, regular inspection by the commissioners. They had already condemned the continued use of the building for that purpose without improvements whose cost was such as to have decided everyone to construct the new asylum at Arlesey! Nevertheless, Mr. Higgins proved to have been correct in his forecast. When the Three Counties committee reported to the Bedford justices in January 1863, it was stated that the new asylum, which had been built to accommodate 504 patients, would be full by the end of that year and that further accommodation would then be necessary.)

At the meeting of Bedfordshire quarter sessions in January 1862 it was reported that a temporary loan had been raised on the county rate from the London Life Office towards the cost of completion of the Three Counties. The sum of £3,000 was due to be repaid by midsummer, but there was no possibility that a sale could be effected by then.

Mr. Higgins now saw "no hope of selling the old asylum as it stood, although there might be parties who would give a certain sum for it and were waiting for it to be offered by auction".

Mr. Starey advised the court to "wait a bit longer as he believed that there were some speculators who would come forward and make some propositions".

At the next meeting the committee decided to offer the asylum for sale by auction (in one lot) in London. If that were not successful, it was to be offered again, this time in three lots: the main building and the land on which it stood, and the two wings with their land on each side. On July 8th 1862, two years after the Bedford asylum had been emptied of patients, it was announced that Messrs. Farebrother and Co. had put it up for auction in one lot.

The sum realised by the sale was £5,000, and the purchasers had until Michaelmas to complete the transaction.

Then came the reckoning; £5,000 was now owed to the London Life Office, £1,900 to Messrs. Barnard, the bankers, and £125 (2½%) to Farebrother and Co. Furthermore, the bills for advertising had not yet arrived. (The original cost of the Bedford asylum had been £13,000.)

John Harvey took the opportunity to remind the committee that when he had proposed additions to the old asylum rather than going to the expense of building a new one, "the notion had been opposed by Mr. Orlebar, Colonel [W. B.] Higgins and Mr. [W. H.] Whitbread". And that, said Mr. Harvey, was the origin of the new asylum.

The implication that he and the other two magistrates carried most of the responsibility for the deficit produced an outraged response from Mr. Orlebar. He did not recall, he said, "having been instrumental in promoting the new asylum and objected to having Mr. Harvey's pet-child thrust upon him".

Mr. Harvey replied that if he had happened to have a copy of the *Bedfordshire Times* on him "he could show Mr. Orlebar what he had said on that occasion"; an expression of confidence in that journal's accuracy which must have put the reporter on his mettle:

"... The discussion got rather bewildering as well as amusing, when Sir J. Burgoyne said he might quote some remarks made in another place which seemed to apply to the present discussion – 'There is nothing in the world more calculated to lead to no result whatever than a discussion about what "he said" and "I said" because it is quite certain that no two people would agree as to what was said by another (laughter)'."

The subject was then dropped, but only until the meeting in October 1862, when the Clerk of the Peace reported that the purchasers, the British Land Company (a firm of developers), had accepted the title and completion of the purchase.

The cudgels were next taken up by Lieutenant-Colonel W. B. Higgins on behalf of the outraged trio – so far from being favourable to the project for building a costly asylum, he had steadily withheld his support, he maintained.

John Harvey replied that he "had no idea that a joke spoken in an undertone would have given rise to serious discussion". However, he repeated his assertion that Higgins, Orlebar and Whitbread had been the first to suggest a new asylum. *He*, Harvey, had brought forward a plan to extend the old building; *they* had objected. Although he had disapproved of the proceedings of the committee for the new building ... he rejoiced that it had been so carried out. So far from wishing to share the responsibility, he gloried in the part he had taken and should reflect with satisfaction on it to his dying day.

"After a few remarks from the chairman," wrote the reporter, "the discussion dropped, the merits of the question being left in about the same position as they were previously."

By January 1863, the loans had been repaid following the sale of the old asylum and the justices felt able to leave it to history to decide between the disputants.

Theed Pearse, the clerk of the peace, had undertaken certain legal work in connection with the sale in his professional capacity (he was a solicitor) and when pressed, had submitted a bill for out-of-pocket expenses amounting to £7.12s.9d. The committee regarded that as quite inadequate and proposed to add a gratuity of £20, but Mr. Pearse was politely adamant and would accept only the expenses.

The chairman, Thomas Charles Higgins, now brought the justices back to earth (literally) by reminding them of the fact that the asylum cemetery had not been part of the sale; it contained no fewer than 498 bodies, and they were still responsible for them. Furthermore, no right of way had been reserved for access.

Mr. Higgins said that he had visited the cemetery and was appalled at the vandalism that had taken place – he was surprised at the carelessness with which some people regarded it. Something had to be done to prevent further desecration.

The justices agreed; the first step was to protect the graves so that nobody could get to them. The question of a right of way was to be explored and an estimate obtained of the cost of moving the bodies to the Bedford cemetery. Finally, they needed to be reassured as to the legality of selling consecrated ground [see p. 86].

The matter was referred to what was described as the "old committee", which recommended that the bodies should not be removed. A wall on the eastern side, which had never been completed, was to be made good. The gates were to be secured and lined with sheet iron. As for access – it appeared that the new owners were building a road along the western side of the cemetery. When that had been finished, it was recommended that the gates be removed so as to open on to the new road for more convenient access.

The British Land Company willingly agreed to the proposal, and as a further gesture, their clerk of works wrote in support of a plea from Mr. Ambridge, the former gardener to the asylum, who had worked there for more than 25 years. On one occasion, Ambridge said, he had been "kicked by a patient and received much injury". He asked the court "to allow him to have the cemetery and some other privileges"; he was "much attached to the spot and if the county would do something for him he might be able to get a home there".

The clerk of works made a more modest suggestion: that the old pump house and a piece of ground be purchased for him. The matter was referred to the old committee, and it, the future of the Bedford asylum and of its cemetery were no longer the concern of quarter sessions.

The justices moved on, no doubt with relief, to consider the affairs of Bedford County Gaol and its inmates, for whose management they still retained responsibility. And their former patients also moved on; into the next era – that of the large mental hospitals.

Another 100 years were to pass before they, too, declined and the patients were destined to return into the communities from which their predecessors had originally been extracted.

In the 48 years of its existence, the Bedford asylum had admitted large numbers of the mentally sick poor; many of them would otherwise have roamed the streets and country lanes until they were arrested for being without visible means of support, and were sent to prison or the workhouse. Others might have landed up in private asylums, where conditions, in the late 18th and early 19th century were in some cases worse than either.

Many patients had been discharged, as being now of sound mind and fit to resume their place in the community. (The term "cured" was not applied to their condition as was the case with the patients discharged from the Infirmary; that would have implied that the treatment they had received was directly responsible for their improvement – they were described as "recovered".)

During the first 30 years of its existence the treatment at the asylum was mainly custodial, and little different from that accorded to the inmates of the county gaol or of the workhouse. Although the York Retreat had been founded in 1796, it was not until 1813, a year after the Bedford asylum had been opened, that Samuel Tuke published his account of the "moral" treatment of the insane there, a report which was in due course to exercise a profound influence on their management. The approach of the Bedfordshire justices was pragmatic; they were guided by whatever precedents were available and at the time, physical methods of restraint, the chains and straps and handcuffs, were a commonplace. As Bedfordshire got off the mark so quickly, for reasons which have been described earlier, the asylum and its true begetter, Samuel Whitbread, acquired a reputation for expertise in the field.

The governing committee of visiting justices had, to all appearances, full confidence in the way that their charges were treated by the governor and keepers. But official minutes do not, of course, tell the whole story, and on occasion the seemingly smooth surface of events was broken by the reefs and shoals that lay underneath; the asylum was neither better nor worse than any other in that respect.

Psychiatry, as a medical specialty, did not get under way until after the move to Arlesey (and it had its origins in this country mainly in an association of medical superintendents of the large asylums). The Bedford magistrates relied on their doctors for medical advice, but how far that extended to an understanding of mental illness was not capable of precise definition.

Of the four senior doctors who attended the patients at the Bedford asylum, it was, perhaps, Joseph Thackeray who showed the greatest willingness to comprehend his role in their management, but he was deeply committed to the affairs of the Infirmary,* as well as to his own practice. Furthermore, his death when he was at the height of his career cut short that earlier promise.

John Harris, who served for a longer period than the others, was conscientious and hard working, but there is little evidence that the rather idealistic approach of his original statements was able to survive the practical difficulties faced by the medical superintendent of such an institution.

It was William Denne who, in the end, was landed with all the problems of managing an asylum that was dilapidated, grossly overcrowded and scheduled for closure. With the backing of the commissioners in lunacy and the more enlightened of the visiting justices (such as Henry Littledale), Denne was able to rid the institution of the last traces of physical restraint to which some of the staff had clung for so long.

He and his wife fully earned the praise of the commissioners and of casual visitors and continued the good work when they accompanied the patients in the move to the Three Counties asylum (now Fairfield Hospital).

The visiting magistrates themselves were drawn from a fairly closed circle of Bedfordshire society; wealthy landowners, gentleman farmers, the clergy and a few medical men for the most part. The governors of the Infirmary, and the guardians who ran the House of Industry (later, the Bedford Union) were drawn from a similar group – in some cases the same individuals served on more than one body. Some brought to their visits a special field of expertise: the yield and quality of the asylum farm produce, the quality of the food and drink provided for the patients, or the care of their souls.

---

* See *Private Charity and the Public Purse – op. cit.*

What they possessed in common, though, was experience in the handling of money, and as we have seen, it was the difficulty of financing the necessary expansion of the Bedford asylum to meet a growing social need which enforced its closure. Ironically enough, the same problems – increasing numbers of homeless, mentally-aberrant people crowding the prisons and workhouses or at large in the community had resulted in the legislation that brought it into existence in the first place.

The answer was to build even bigger institutions; the Three Counties asylum, for example. One hundred years later, there came the move towards "care in the community", which was the subject of a comprehensive review by Michael Shepherd in the *British Medical Journal* (September 9th 1989). He quotes Richard Titmuss, who wrote, in 1963:

> "To scatter the mentally ill in the community before we have made adequate provision for them is not a solution . . . we are drifting into a situation in which, by shifting the emphasis from the institution to the community – a trend which, in principle and with qualifications, we all applaud – we are transferring the care of the mentally ill from trained staff to untrained or ill-equipped staff or no staff at all."

"Experiment, evaluation and comparison are needed," says Shepherd, "if we are to turn Titmuss's fictions of yesterday into the facts of tomorrow".

References

The main primary sources of material concerning the Bedford asylum are held at the County Record Office (CRO); they are catalogued under the general heading . . . LB.

There are too many to allow individual citation of references in the text without unacceptable clutter, but the records which have been consulted include the following:

1. Minutes of the asylum 1812-1860	LB1/1-11;
2. Visitors' reports 1822-1860	LB2/3
3. Lists of patients, admissions, discharges, medical reports etc....................................	LB3/(various);
4. Medical and visiting surgeon's journals..	LB3/16-20;
5. General expenditure, account books	LB5/1-5;
6. Inventories 1834-1843	LB6/1-4;
7. Additions and alterations 1847	LB7/1, also LBP/3 and PL;
8. Miscellaneous, including correspondence	LB7/12-16, 19;
9. Misc. papers 1812-1852	LBP/1, 7;
10. Minutes of the Bedfordshire Quarter Sessions...	QS/(various);
11. The Whitbread correspondence	W1/136-180;
12. Report of the select committee of the House of Commons on the state of lunatics, 1807..	British Library

The minute book of the joint committee for the Three Counties Asylum is retained in the archives at Fairfield Hospital and is unclassified.

The files of the *Bedford Record* and of *The Bedfordshire Times* have also been consulted, particularly with regard to the sale of the asylum and its aftermath.

Bibliography

BYNUM, W. F.; Psychiatry in its historical context – in *Handbook of Psychiatry*, (Ed. Shepherd, M. and Zangwill, O. L.), Vol. 1, Routledge: 1988.

BYNUM, W. F., SHEPHERD, M. and PORTER, R. (Eds.); *The Anatomy of Madness*, Vol. 3, Cambridge University Press: 1983.

CASHMAN, BERNARD; *Private Charity and the Public Purse*, N. Beds. Health Authority: 1988.

CIRKET, ALAN F.; In the shadow of the Wings, *Beds. Magazine*, XV p. 278.

COLE, DENNIS; Satirical prints of Whitbread in the British Museum, in *Apollo*: October 1973.

COLLET-WHITE, JAMES; "Such as are distressed and afflicted in minde", *Beds. Magazine,* XVII p. 25.

COLWIN, HOWARD (Ed.); *Biographical Dictionary of British Architects,* London, John Murray: 1978.

FULFORD, ROGER; *Samuel Whitbread – a study in opposition, Macmillan, London: 1967.*

JONES, KATHLEEN; *A history of the mental health services*: London, Routledge and Kegan Paul: 1972.

HUNTER, R. and MACALPINE, I. (Eds.); *Three hundred years of psychiatry*, London, Oxford University Press: 1963.

PICKSTONE, JOHN; *Social History of Medicine*, Vol. 2, 2, p. 198.

PORTER, ROY; *Mind-forg'd manacles*, Athlone Press: 1987.

SCULL, A.; *Museums of madness*, London: Allen Lane: 1979.

STOCKDALE, ERIC; *A Study of Bedford Prison 1660-1877*, Bedfordshire Historical Record Society Vol. 56 (1977).

STOCKDALE, ERIC; *Law and Order in Georgian Bedfordshire,* Bedfordshire Historical Record Society Vol. 61.

Appendices

APPENDIX I

September 4th 1815, Dr. Joseph Thackeray to Lord St. John:

"My Lord

Since the receipt of your Lordship's letter on the subject of the Asylum, I have considered of the means best-calculated to fulfil the intentions of the magistrates in regard to the medical department of that institution.

"The office which it is proposed to establish is one requiring some ability and much patient attention for its due execution. The present state of the house in which there are but few subjects under medical treatment may perhaps have led to the idea that little occasion exists for the establishment of such a department. Were this state a permanent condition of the House the conclusion would be just; but it should be regarded wholly an accidental one depending on the infancy of the institution.

"The asylum is at present filled chiefly with patients whose disorders from their long-standing discourage every hope of benefit from medical exertion. In the progress however of time recent cases of derangement will be continually presenting themselves, when much encouragement will be offered for the active interference of Art. That its endeavours are not altogether fruitless, a reference to the reports of the house will perhaps satisfy your Lordship.

"As the incurableness of mental disorders is a notion very generally received even in the medical world, and one which seems to have met with your Lordship's assent, I hope to be excused for expressing my sentiments as decidedly at variance with this opinion.

"Daily experience teaches me that a costive state of the body, a disordered state of the stomach, and a pregnant condition of the womb are capable of inducing temporary melancholy, and great irregularity of moral action; and little difference is, I think, to be observed between the ravings of the drunkard, and the paroxysms of the maniac, beyond the length of their duration.

"The influence of these circumstances upon the mind prove its dependence and subjection to physical agents; and if physical agents can thus induce moral disorder, it is reasonable to presume that moral disorder may be corrected by physical agents.

"Mental diseases may, I think, be classed in a general way under three heads – maniacal, melancholic and nervous. The first and second classes are generally connected with diseased action of the body – mania being connected with morbid action of the brain, and melancholia with morbid action of some of the abdominal viscera. These two genera are not unfrequently combined. The third class seems to depend on peculiar states of the nervous, as the two others do on certain conditions of the sanguineous system.

"If there be any foundation for this classification of mental disorders, great encouragement is I think held out for placing a lunatic asylum on the footing of a medical institution.

"I ought to apologise to your Lordship for this trespass upon your time; but as you were pleased to invite me to the discussion in your letter, I have ventured to avail myself of the indulgence.

"With respect to a suitable officer for the situation in question, I have had some difficulty in fulfilling the wishes of the magistrates; as the office does not offer those inducements which similar appointments hold out at general medical institutions.

"A salary of fifty pounds with board seems to be the lowest sum that could be offered to a respectable young man for discharging the duties of house-apothecary and secretary to the institution.

"Your Lordship and the rest of the magistrates would of course be pleased to make such arrangements as would not require the officer to have a common-table with the governor and matron.

"I have the honor to remain, my Lord
"Yr Obedt Servant
Joseph Thackeray"

APPENDIX II

Letter from John Harris: to the magistrates:

"Lunatic Asylum March 2nd.1829

"Gentlemen

"In obedience to your commands I beg leave to lay before you a few observations relative to an improved medical and moral treatment of the patients confined in this establishment, but I cannot do this without expressing the diffidence I feel in giving an opinion on a subject of which I have yet so little knowledge.

"It is the opinion of most modern authors who have written on insanity, that it, in almost all cases results from some corporeal disease, and that we must cure the disease of the mind by remedies applied to the body. I do not think that our attention should be exclusively devoted to the one or the other but that whilst we attempt the restoration of the general health by physical, we should correct the aberrations of the mind by moral agents; and as a means of fulfilling both these indications I know of none equal to some rational employment, which will at once benefit the body and by degrees call forth the reasoning properties of the mind.

"I would therefore with deference recommend that every patient who is capable and can be trusted should have some occupation suited to his former habits, taking care to avoid those exciting causes which had proved prejudicial; and, as most of the patients confined in the asylum have been brought up in agricultural pursuits, I think they might be beneficially employed in the cultivation of land and in the care of cows sheep, pigs &c. and in the case of mechanics they might work at their various trades such as carpentering, tailoring, painting, shoemaking &c.

"How far attention has been paid to these points we may judge when we reflect on the manner in which lunatics have, for too long a time, been treated – shut up within the walls of a prison with the same objects continually around them, without any change or incident to excite attention and break the train of diseased imagination or call back erring reason to her healthy course without any inducements to take the exercise necessary for bodily health, shut out from all the soothing attentions of kindred friends and without anyone to quiet by kind treatment their troubled minds. Can it then be any wonder that ideas, cherished from day to day and week to week in the same monotonous existence, should become permanently fixed, and the once curable lunatic become a confirmed madman to drag out a wretched life until death shall terminate his sufferings?

"With regard to the treatment of patients from the ranks of society superior to paupers and who have been accustomed to look to amusements as a means of passing some of their time I would recommend the perusal of some entertaining and instructive books on history and travels, as well as the current news of the day, which would not only beguile their tedious hours, but would keep alive an association with the world and prevent their falling into that state of apathy so frequently observed, and should they be restored to their homes, they will not feel that their life had been such a blank as to a knowledge of passing events during their absence from society.

"I think that the effect of some instrumental music should be tried, and perhaps a hand-organ would answer this purpose.

"As a remedy to improve the bodily health of the insane I believe that bathing holds one of the first ranks, and I would strongly recommend that all lunatic asylums should have proper warm, and cold baths.

"Finally as a means of putting the above ideas to the test I beg respectfully to recommend that such a quantity of land be cultivated as would supply almost constant employment for the patients and for the pasturage of more cows in whose care some would find an agreeable occupation and the house would thus be supplied with a sufficient quantity of milk and butter.

"I would recommend the erection of a carpenter's shop, which might also be adapted to the pursuit of other mechanical occupations.

"Having given these my humble opinions I beg to leave it to your judgment how far they are worthy of your consideration.

I have the honor to be
Gentlemen
Your obedt. humble servant
J.Harris"

APPENDIX III

Springfield House Private Asylum (1837-1962):
by Nigel Lutt, archivist, Bedfordshire County Record Office

Springfield House, which opened in Kempston in 1837, was the only purpose-built private asylum in Bedfordshire. The county asylum in Ampthill Road had admitted both pauper and private patients but with the passage of the new Poor Law Act in 1834, an increase in the number of pauper patients was expected, with further pressure on the rates which provided the finances. John Harris, the medical superintendent, proposed to open a private asylum on his own account, and the Committee of Visiting Justices agreed that only pauper patients would be admitted to the county institution.

In the summer of 1835 John Harris began looking for a site for the new asylum. He approached Thomas Bennett, the Duke of Bedford's estate agent, and asked if His Grace would lease him the site occupied by St. Leonard's farmhouse near the junction of Ampthill Road and London Road, Bedford. Bennett was doubtful. The value of the surrounding building plots would be reduced if the asylum was built too near to Bedford town centre. Would Harris consider a site adjacent to the county asylum in Ampthill Road? "To this site he has no objection," wrote Bennett on July 7th. However by mid-August John Harris had changed his mind. "Mr. Harris says there is an insuperable objection to it by being so close to the County Asylum," Bennett noted drily on the 18th. ". . . between the patients' yard there would only be a narrow close bounded by a brick wall and that the language of many of the patients is such that he could not place his private patients within hearing. . . ."

Harris eventually found a site on the north side of Elstow Road, Kempston – safely out of earshot of the county asylum! Thomas Gwyn Elger, an architect who had designed the treadmills at Bedford Prison, was commissioned to draw up the plans. Building work began in the spring of 1836 and in March 1837 the asylum was licensed to receive thirty patients, each of whom paid a guinea a week in fees. On April 28th Springfield Asylum opened and the private patients were transferred from the county asylum to the new buildings in Elstow Road. The asylum had cost John Harris over £2,000 to build.

The Springfield House Visitors' book provides interesting glimpses of conditions in the asylum in the nineteenth century. Restraint of the patients by belts, muffs and strait-jackets was commonplace in the early years. The Commissioners in Lunacy recommended in February 1851 that the stables and chains attached to some of the bedsteads should be removed. John Harris was unwilling to comply, being ". . . unable to dispense with restraint". By the 1870s seclusion was increasingly used instead of restraint and padded rooms were built in 1894 off the main dormitories.

On a lighter note we read that patients were encouraged to meet in the evenings for cards, music and reading. During the day patients could walk escorted around the grounds and some visited Elstow church on Sundays. Food was apparently of good quality. On April 12th 1859 the commissioners noted that there were "abundant portions . . . of roast pork, two vegetables and rhubarb pudding".

In 1855, Springfield was licensed to admit ten extra patients and the clothes room in the staff block was changed into a dormitory to accommodate them. These and other alterations were approved by the commissioners, who also recommended that ". . . the walls of the airing yards be lowered as they have a depressing aspect".

John Harris died in 1861 and was succeeded by his son Henry as resident surgeon. Henry was in failing health and died suddenly in 1878. His mother Sophia, who worked as matron, wanted to continue running the asylum, but the commissioners considered that "the licence ought not to be permanently renewed to her unless she introduces . . . some approved medical man who will be resident".

In June 1879 the asylum was sold privately to Dr. David Bower, a Scotsman who had worked at Saughton Hall private asylum in Edinburgh. By this time overcrowding had become a problem at Springfield. The asylum was changed to admit forty-seven patients; new wings containing dormitories and dayrooms were added in 1890-95 and a new dining room in 1912. The energetic Dr. Bower also introduced the "employment" system and patients were encouraged to do gardening or work at embroidery. An advertisement of 1885 lists billiards, tennis, boating and carriage-drives among the recreations.

Dr. Bower died in 1929 after 50 years in charge of Springfield Asylum. His son Cedric became medical superintendent. A combination of rising costs, falling applications and the problems of recruiting adequate staff led to his decision to close the asylum at the end of August 1962, and most of the patients were transferred to St. Andrew's Hospital at Northampton. In 1963 Springfield Asylum was demolished to make way for the expansion of Kempston New Town. Henderson Way, Fearnley Crescent and Whittingstall Avenue now occupy the site but "Springfield Cottage" built for Dr. David Bower when he married in 1888 still stands in Spring Road, Kempston.

APPENDIX IV

The Actual Cost of the Patients in the Bedford Lunatic Asylum during the year 1853

Names of Counties and Unions		Collecting number of Days Patients were maintained	Actual cost to the Asylum at 7-10¾			Sums received on account thereof including balance from last year			Balance due from the Asylum			Balance due to the Asylum		
Albans St.	Union	2634	148	11	1	135	0	2		10	11	13	10	11
Ampthill	Union	6611	372	17	1	364	8	3				8	8	10
Barnet	Union	365	20	11	9	14	19	.				5	12	9
Bedford County		475	26	15	10	21	15	1				5	0	9
Bedford	Union	13891	783	8	9	760	11	8				22	17	1
Berkhamstead	Union	1683	94	18	5	94	12	6				.	5	11
Biggleswade	Union	5118	288	13	.	285	7	4				3	5	8
Bishop Stortford	Union	4662	267	18	7	256	17	7				6	1	–
Buntingford	Union	2535	142	19	5	138	1	8				4	17	9
Caxton	Union	365	20	11	9	19	17	7					14	2
Edmonton	Union	1095	61	15	2	59	12	9				2	2	5
Hatfield	Union	3998	225	9	8	218	13	5				6	16	3
Hemel Hempstead	Union	3285	185	5	5	171	12	6				13	12	11
Hertford	County	365	20	11	9	19	17	7					14	2
Hertford	Union	4963	279	18	2	271	2	9				8	15	5
Hitchin	Union	7924	446	18	1	435	16	.				11	2	1
Huntingdon	County	730	41	3	5	39	15	.				1	8	5
Huntingdon	Union	5483	309	4	8	307	8	9				1	15	11
Ives Saint	Union	6459	364	5	7	356	19	6				7	6	1
Leighton Buzzard	Union	1159	65	7	4	63	1	11				2	5	5
Luton	Union	5886	331	19	3	329	0	10				2	18	5
Monmouth	Union	10		11	3		11	3				–	–	–
Neots St.	Union	4076	229	17	8	227	8	.				2	9	8
Peterborough	Union	917	51	14	1	47	16	.				3	18	4
Royston	Union	365	20	11	9	19	17	7					14	2
Ware	Union	3186	179	13	9	174	7	3				5	6	6
Watford	Union	6060	341	15	7	318	18	4				22	17	3
Welwyn	Union	724	40	16	8	39	17	2					19	6
Woburn	Union	4036	228	15	1	220	14	7				8	0	6
		99080	5586	0	3	5414	2	0				173	18	3

1

Receipts and Payments

ON ACCOUNT OF THE

BEDFORD LUNATIC ASYLUM,

IN THE YEAR ENDING 31st, DECEMBER, 1853.

RECEIPTS.

FROM SALES.	£.	s.	d.	£	s.	d.
Produce of Garden and Farm	222	6	2			
Sundries, old stores, bone, &c.	8	4	10			
				230	11	0

From Unions and Parishes in the United Counties of Bedford, Hertford, and Huntingdon, and the Borough of Bedford, viz.:

COUNTY OF BEDFORD.	£.	s.	d.	£	s.	d.
Ampthill Union	381	16	1			
Bedford Union	753	9	3			
Biggleswade Union	313	17	0			
Leighton Buzzard Union	60	7	11			
Luton Union	327	15	3			
Woburn Union	220	14	0			
COUNTY OF HERTFORD.						
Alban's St. Union	144	12	5			
Barnet Union	14	19	0			
Berkhampstead Union	99	12	4			
Bishop Stortford Union	253	19	1			
Buntingford Union	138	0	8			
Edmonton Union	74	8	6			
Hatfield Union	219	13	11			
Hemel Hempstead Union	178	1	7			
Hertford Union	271	12	9			
Hitchin Union	432	3	11			
Royston Union	19	3	8			
Ware Union	192	4	5			
Watford Union	329	16	3			
Welwyn Union	39	15	2			
Carried forward	£4466	3	2	230	11	0

2

				£.	s.	d.	£.	s.	d.
Brought forward				4466	3	2	230	11	0
COUNTY OF HUNTINGDON.									
Caxton Union				19	17	7			
Huntingdon Union				298	3	9			
St. Ives Union				352	19	0			
St. Neots Union				218	13	5			
Peterborough Union				47	2	6			
							5402	19	5
From the County, Liberty, and Borough Treasurers, in the United Counties and Borough for Vagrants, Paupers, and Criminal Lunatics, respectively, viz.:									
Albans, St., Liberty				37	7	11			
Bedford, County				92	0	9			
Hertford, County				57	5	11			
Huntingdon, County				63	18	8			
							250	13	3
From the following Counties for the excess in the weekly sums paid for Criminal Lunatics, chargeable to Parishes beyond the sums charged for the Maintenance of Patients in this Asylum,—(16 & 17 Vict. cap. 97, s. 42.)									
Bedford, County				20	12	10			
Hertford, County				20	12	10			
							41	5	8
From out-Counties and non-contributory Districts, viz.:									
Monmouth Union				5	7	6			
Oxford County				1	8	0			
							6	15	6
From the County of Bedford									
For ordinary Repairs							115	11	6
From the United Counties and Borough, their respective proportions of excess of Contract for Building New Chapel, Washhouse, and Laundry, viz.:									
Bedford, County	10	1	8						
„ Borough	1	0	2	11	1	10			
Hertford, County				16	12	8			
Huntingdon, County				6	3	7			
							33	18	1
From the United Counties and Borough, their respective proportions of cost of erecting Cemetery Wall, viz.:									
Bedford, County	28	7	10						
„ Borough	2	16	9	31	4	7			
Hertford, County				46	16	11			
Huntingdon, County				17	3	5			
							95	4	11
Total Receipts							£6176	19	4

3

PAYMENTS.

PROVISIONS.				£.	s.	d.	£.	s.	d.
Arrowroot,...56 ℔s. @ 1s. and carriage 1s.				2	17	0			
Bacon, 240 ℔s. @ 6½d. & 7¼d, ℘ ℔.				6	16	4			
Baking,				0	19	4			
Beer, 14366 galls. @ 6¾d. ℘ gall. viz.									
Malt, 969 bus. @ 6s. 6d. & 6s. 11½d. ℘ bus.	326	10	6						
Hops, 1131 ℔s. @ 11d. & 1. 4d. ℘ ℔	60	5	11						
Brewer, ...68 days, @ 3s. ℘ day	10	4	0						
				397	0	5			
Bread.........30497 loaves, @ 4½d. to 8d. ℘ loaf				721	18	10			
Buns,				1	15	6			
Butter, ...3836 ℔s. @ 88s. 8d. to 91s. ℘ cwt. and 11d. & 1s. ℘ ℔...				156	8	4			
Cheese,......9358 ℔s. @ 60s. to 68s. ℘ cwt.				268	17	1			
Coffee, 300 ℔s. @ 11d. ℘ ℔. & carriage				14	2	6			
Currants,......896 ℔s. @ 52s. & 60s. ℘ cwt.				22	12	0			
Fish				0	13	0			
Flour,......43 sacks, @ 33s. & 40s. ℘ sack				82	10	0			
Fruit				0	5	0			
Meat, 42862 ℔s. @ 4½d. to 5½d. ℘ ℔.				936	16	6			
Milk,...2949 gals. @ 4¾d. ℘ gal.....				58	7	3			
Oatmeal, 11 sacks, @ 32s. & 32s. 6d. ℘ sack				17	18	9			
Peas, 24 bus. @ 8s. & 8s. 6d. ℘ bus.				9	16	0			
* Potatoes, ...50 bus. @ 3s. ℘ bus...				7	10	0			
Raisins, 472 ℔s. @ 4½d. & 5d. ℘ ℔.				9	6	4			
Rice, 506 ℔s. @ 1¾d. to 5d. ℘ ℔. ...				3	7	7			
Sugar (loaf) ...159¾ ℔s. @ 5½d. ℘ ℔.	3	13	3						
„ (moist) 3699 ℔s. @ 37 s. & 37s. 4d. ℘ cwt.	61	8	0						
				65	1	3			
Carried forward.....							£2784	19	0

* The cost of the Vegetables consumed from the produce of the Garden during the year amounts to £107 : 10 : 0, and has been calculated in the cost per head, per week, accordingly.

4

	£.	s.	d.	£.	s.	d.
PROVISIONS *(continued)*						
Brought forward	2784	19	0			
Tea, ...347 lbs. @ 3s. 8d. & 3s. 4d. ℔ lb. and carriage....................	61	2	6			
Vinegar, mustard, pepper, salt and spices......	8	19	0			
Wine, 3 doz. british, @ 20s. ℔ doz.	3	0	0			
				2858	0	6

Note—In calculating the cost per head per week, £553 : 16 : 11¼, for maintenance of household is deducted from this sum, and added to Salaries and Wages.

	£.	s.	d.	£.	s.	d.
NECESSARIES.						
Candles,...144 lbs. @ 5s. 3d. & 7s. 6d. ℔ doz.	3	7	6			
Coals, ...275¼ tons, @ 18s. 9d. to 21s. 9d. ℔ ton	297	6	11			
Gas,......256,300 cubic feet @ 5s. 6d. ℔ thousand feet	70	9	7			
Soap,...66 cwt. 2 qrs. 24 lbs. @ 34s. to 49s. ℔ cwt.	136	8	6			
Soda, ...38 cwt. 2 qrs. 15 lbs. 6d. 6s. and 6s. 9d. ℔ cwt.	12	16	6			
Starch and blue	3	2	4			
Washing	35	8	6			
				558	19	10
CLOTHING.						
Braces and gloves.........................	3	17	3			
Caps	9	10	10			
Calico	21	17	8			
Flannel	31	18	9			
Fustian	26	1	8			
Handkerchiefs	7	17	11			
Jean	3	19	1			
Lindsey woolsey	20	0	0			
Linen...	5	2	7			
Muslin	3	2	0			
Pilot cloth....................................	47	17	3			
Pocketing	3	10	0			
Print	20	4	0			
Shirting cloth	21	4	4			
Shoemaker..................	130	14	5			
Stays	24	17	6			
Stockings	38	3	6			
Tailor..	39	8	4			
Carried forward	£459	7	1	3417	0	4

5

				£.	s.	d.	£.	s.	d
CLOTHING, *(continued,)*									
Brought forward				459	7	1	3417	0	4
Thread, tape, cottons, worsted, buttons, &c				31	17	9			
Wrappering				8	18	3			
							500	3	1
SURGERY AND DISPENSARY.									
Drugs				17	5	0			
Surgical Instruments				6	11	0			
Wine and Spirits				24	8	3			
							47	19	3
SALARIES AND WAGES.									
Superintendent				150	0	0			
Resident Medical Officer	100	0	0						
Gratuity	45	0	0						
				145	0	0			
Clerk to Visitors	100	0	0						
Gratuity	20	0	0						
				120	0	0			
Chaplain				80	0	0			
Matron				36	5	0			
Assistant Matron				18	10	0			
Storekeeper and Chief Ward Attendant				33	16	0			
Nine Male Ward Attendants, @ 9s. and 11s. per week each				213	11	6			
Gardener				31	8	0			
Seven Female Ward Attendants, @ £8. £10. and £12. ℘ annum each				64	13	6			
Two Laundressess				22	18	4			
Sempstress				14	0	0			
Female Nurse				13	0	0			
Cook				12	12	0			
Housemaid				7	1	6			
Kitchen-maid				8	0	0			
Porter				12	7	0			
Stoker (10 weeks)				2	10	0			
Shaver				14	10	0			
Chapel Clerk, (1½-year)				8	15	0			
Extra Nurses, Assistants, &c.				3	16	0			
							*1007	13	10
Carried forward							£4972	16	6

* In calculating the cost per head per week, £553 : 16 : 11¼, the charges for the Maintenance of the household is added to this sum.

6

	£.	s.	d.	£.	s.	d.
Brought forward				4972	13	6
MISCELLANEOUS.						
Baskets, and mending same	7	8	8			
Belts	0	13	0			
Blacking	0	19	8			
Black lead	0	7	10			
Books	4	1	0			
Brushes, mops, &c, ...	38	19	2			
Chimney sweeper	4	15	3			
Clock repairing	0	4	0			
Clothes pegs	0	14	6			
Combs	4	2	0			
Corks	0	7	6			
Cricket and foot balls, &c	2	6	0			
Cooperage	7	7	3			
Earthenware	14	3	10			
Easter offering	0	10	0			
Expenses of Meeting at Hitchin......	1	16	2			
Expenses of recovering Patients......	2	7	6			
Glazing and plumbing	18	5	8			
Gravestones	0	9	0			
Hearthstones	0	18	0			
Insurance	14	7	6			
Ironmongery	28	13	1			
Marking ink	1	0	0			
Matches	1	0	0			
Music for Patient's ball	0	15	0			
Olive oil	2	7	6			
Patent sheeting	1	10	0			
Postage and carriage	13	0	8			
Post Office fee	1	1	0			
Posting bills	0	10	0			
Rates and taxes *(a)*	41	0	4			
Rope	1	2	5			
Sand	5	17	1			
Snuff and tobacco	39	8	6			
Stationery, printing, and advertisements	40	5	6			
Seraphine for Chapel	3	0	0			
Spectacles	1	4	6			
Straw	45	6	6			
Sundries	5	3	11			
Turner	1	3	5			
				358	12	11
Carried forward				5331	9	5

(a) Two improvement rates are included.

7

				£.	s.	d.	£.	s.	d.
Brought forward							5331	9	5
FUNERAL EXPENSES.									
Ordinary repairs, account for coffins, (a)							10	10	0
REMOVAL OF PATIENTS.									
Expenses of removals (a)							0	14	6
FURNITURE, BEDDING, FIXTURES, AND FITTINGS.									
Bed ticking				8	9	10			
Blankets				41	18	10			
Carver and Gilder				0	8	0			
Furniture Check				1	10	3			
Gas fittings				1	18	11			
Hot water apparatus				119	3	9			
Ironmonger				20	6	0			
Rugs				17	1	6			
Sacking				5	16	0			
Sheeting				67	9	7			
Building Account, viz.—									
Carpenter	53	19	4						
Bricklayer	6	19	10						
Smith	17	10	8						
				78	9	10			
							362	12	6
BUILDING ACCOUNT, ORDINARY REPAIRS.									
Barker John, plumber				0	10	1			
Bevan Benjamin, timber				9	7	2			
Brown John, bricks and lime				10	2	7			
Carling Thomas, plumber				2	2	8			
Conquest Josiah, carpenter				10	3	0			
Francis Samuel, bricks and cement				7	5	7			
Hands Richard, carpenter				28	18	3			
Hinde William, plumber				18	17	1			
Howard Jas. and F. ironmongers				2	8	10			
Kilpin Wm. W., ditto				2	18	0			
Millington Thomas, oils and colors				13	0	1			
Morton Thomas, ironmonger				17	13	10			
Palgrave C. F., for paint brushes				1	3	6			
Salmon W. E., plan of estate				5	5	0			
Slater John, bricklayer				22	4	8			
Steward, as per day book for sundries				28	2	0			
Tacchi Anthony, carver and gilder				0	8	6			
Carried forward				£180	10	10	5705	6	5

(a) These sums have been added to the charges for maintenance, &c, of the respective Patients, for whom they were incurred.

8

		£.	s.	d.	£.	s.	d.
BUILDING ACCOUNT, ETC., *(continued)*							
Brought forward		180	10	10	5705	6	5
Walker, George, for timber		7	16	4			
Williams Wm. ironmonger............		4	3	1			
Wing J. T., stone and cement		0	11	8			
		193	1	11			
Less funeral expenses, transferred	10 10 0						
Furniture, fixtures and fittings transferred.	78 9 10						
		88	19	10			
					104	2	1
MAINTENANCE OF CRIMINAL LUNATICS.							
Dr. Finch, for Maintenance of Nine Patients, from 21st Dec. 1852, to 21st Dec. 1853, ...					271	16	0
GARDEN AND FARM.							
Orders on Treasurer at various times during the year					141	13	3
Total Payments..........................					£6222	17	9

9 STATEMENT OF RECEIPTS AND PAYMENTS ON ACCOUNT OF THE BEDFORD LUNATIC ASYLUM,

Between the 1st of January, and the 31st of December, 1853.

Receipts.

	£.	s.	d.
To Balance in Steward's hands, Dec. 31, 1852...	50	0	0
Receipts under the following heads, *viz:*—			
PAGE.			
Sales.—Produce of Garden and Farm, and Sundries, by Steward	230	11	0
Unions and Parishes in the United Counties of Bedford, Hertford, and Huntingdon, and the Borough of Bedford........................	5402	19	5
County and Borough Treasurers, in united Counties and Borough	250	13	3
Counties of Bedford, and Hertford, excess paid for Maintenance of Criminal Patients chargeable to Parishes (16 & 17 Vict. cap. 97, s. 42.)	41	5	8
Out Counties and non-contributory Districts	6	15	6
County of Bedford, for ordinary repairs......	115	11	6
United Counties and Borough, their respective proportions of the excess of Contract for New Chapel, Wash-house, and Laundry	33	18	1
Also for cost of erecting Cemetery Wall ...	95	4	11
	6226	19	4
Balance due to Treasurer, Dec. 31, 1853,	478	6	11
	£6705	6	3

SAML. WING,
Clerk to the Committee of Visitors

Payments.

	£.	s.	d.
By Balance due to Treasurer, Dec. 31st, 1852...	427	5	6
„ Balance due to Mr. Matthews, ditto	5	3	0
PAGE.			
By Provisions	2858	0	6
„ Necessaries........................	558	19	10
„ Clothing	500	3	1
„ Surgery and Dispensary	47	19	3
„ Salaries and Wages	1007	13	10
„ Miscellaneous........................	358	12	11
„ Funeral Expenses	10	10	0
„ Removal of Patients	0	14	6
„ Furniture, bedding, fixtures, and fittings	362	12	6
„ Building account,—ordinary repairs......	104	2	1
„ Maintenance of Criminal Patients	271	16	0
„ Garden and Farm advances	141	13	3
	6655	6	3
Balance in Steward's hands, Dec. 31st, 1853 ...	50	0	0
	£6705	6	3

14th of February, 1854,
Examined & allowed, } THO. CHA. HIGGINS,
Chairman.

10

ABSTRACT OF THE RECEIPTS & PAYMENTS

For the Year ending

Receipts.

	£.	s.	d.	£.	s.	d.
To Cash for sale of kidney beans ...	0	2	0			
" " manure	4	0	0			
" " onions	9	7	6			
" " pigs	128	15	0			
" " potatoes	8	10	0			
" " sheep	22	7	0			
" " straw...............	11	13	4			
" " wheat	36	4	6			
" " wool	1	6	10			
				222	6	2
Orders on Treasurer at various times during the year				141	13	3
Provisions account, estimated value of the vegetables consumed in the Asylum during the year				107	10	0
Estimated Rent of Garden				6	0	0
Value of Grains, Straw, and Wash consumed on the Garden and Farm, during the year ...				43	17	0
				£521	6	5

STATEMENT OF VALUE OF

On the 31*st of December*,

1852		£.	s.	d.
Dec. 31.	Estimated value of live and dead stock as per last year's account	92	0	0
	Increase 1853, compared with 1852......	124	18	0
		£216	18	0

SAML. WING,
Clerk to the Committee of Visitors.

11

ON ACCOUNT OF THE GARDEN AND FARM.
December 31*st*, 1853.

Payments.

	£.	s.	d.	£.	s.	d.
By Cash for rent, (1 year)	39	18	0			
" pigs	26	0	0			
" sheep	11	2	0			
" garden seeds	2	10	6			
" tares	0	8	0			
" potatoes	8	0	1			
" pollard, &c.	38	5	3			
" peas	8	5	0			
" ironmongery	2	11	0			
" rope	0	6	9			
" thrashing	1	18	10			
" grains	1	7	10			
" wheat	1	0	0			
				141	13	3
Cash to Treasurer at various times, during the year for Sales of produce				222	6	2
Maintenance account—estimated value of the vegetables consumed in the Asylum during the year				107	10	0
Garden account—estimated rent, and value of grains, &c, consumed on the Garden and Farm during the year				49	17	0
				£521	6	5

LIVE AND DEAD STOCK,
1852 *and* 1853, *respectively*,

1853.	£.	s.	d.
Dec. 31. Estimated value of live & dead stock this day, *viz.*—			
Beans	8	8	0
Mangel Wurzel	15	0	0
Manure	20	0	0
Onions	3	0	0
Parsnips	6	0	0
Pigs	60	0	0
Potatoes	90	0	0
Poultry	1	0	0
Sheep	10	10	0
Turnips	3	0	0
	£216	18	0

14*th*, *February*, 1854,
Examined & allowed.

THO. CHA. HIGGINS,
Chairman.

12

THE RATES OF PAYMENT DURING THE YEAR, HAVE BEEN AS FOLLOWS, *viz.*—

	£.	*s.*	*d.*
First Quarter	0	7	6
Second Quarter	0	7	6
Third Quarter	0	8	0
Fourth Quarter	0	7	6
	£1	10	6
Average	0	7	7½

THE ACTUAL WEEKLY COST OF THE PATIENTS AVERAGES AS FOLLOWS, *viz.*—

	s.	*d.*
Provisions	3	4⅜
Necessaries	0	9⅜
Clothing	0	8½
Salaries and Wages	2	2½
Surgery and Dispensary	0	0⅞
Fittings and Furniture	0	6⅛
Other Expenses	0	6¼
	8	2
Less from Miscellaneous Receipts	0	3¼
Net Cost	7	10¾

Average weekly cost of Household... 6s. 2½d.

Daily average of Patients........... 271½

Daily average of Household......... 34

Index